DESIGNING HIV/AIDS INTERVENTION STUDIES

AN OPERATIONS RESEARCH HANDBOOK

Andrew A. Fisher
James R. Foreit

with

John Laing
John Stoeckel
John Townsend

Library of Congress Cataloging-in-Publication Data

Fisher, Andrew A.
    Designing HIV/AIDS intervention studies: an operations research handbook/ Andrew
A. Fisher, James R. Foreit, with John Laing, John Stoeckel, John Townsend.
        p. cm
    Includes bibliographical references.
    ISBN 0-87834-107-2 (pbk)
    1. AIDS (Disease)–Research–Methodology–Handbooks, manuals, etc. 2. Operations
research–Handbooks, manuals, etc. I. Foreit, James R. II. Title.

RA643.8 .F574 2002
616.97'92'072–dc21   2002025266

 This publication was supported by the Horizons Program. Horizons is funded by the Office of
HIV-AIDS, U.S. Agency for International Development, under the terms of Award No. HRN-
A-00-97-00012-00. The opinions expressed herein are those of the authors and do not necessarily
reflect the views of the U.S. Agency for International Development.

Published in May 2002.

Population Council The Population Council is an international, nonprofit, nongovernmental institution that
seeks to improve the wellbeing and reproductive health of current and future generations
around the world and to help achieve a humane, equitable, and sustainable balance
between people and resources. The Council conducts biomedical, social science, and
public health research and helps build research capacities in developing countries. Established in 1952, the
Council is governed by an international board of trustees. Its New York headquarters supports a global network of regional and country offices.

Acknowledgments

This *Handbook* is based on an earlier document written in 1983 with support from the U.S. Agency for International Development, *Handbook for Family Planning Operations Research Design* by Andrew Fisher, John Laing, and John Stoeckel. It was revised in 1991 with the assistance of John Townsend and reprinted in 1998.

This *Handbook* was made possible through support provided by Horizons, a program funded by the Global Bureau of Health/HIV-AIDS, U.S. Agency for International Development, under terms of Award No. HRN-A-00-97-00012-00; and by the Frontiers in Reproductive Health Program, funded by the Office of Population of USAID, under terms of Cooperative Agreement Number HRN-A-00-98-00012-00. The opinions expressed herein are those of the authors and do not necessarily reflect the views of USAID.

The authors are very grateful for the constructive comments they received from many workshop participants and other users of the earlier *Handbook for Family Planning* in Asia, Africa, and Latin America. We are also thankful for the comments, support, and encouragement of colleagues at USAID, cooperating agencies, our partner organizations, international agencies, universities, and the Population Council.

We would especially like to thank our colleagues working on the Population Council's Horizons Program and Frontiers Program for their encouragement and assistance. Also, special thanks to Ellen Weiss, Margaret Dadian, Sherry Hutchinson, Jessica Nicholaides, Amy Ellis, Kathy Keler, and Sharon Schultz for editorial, design, formatting, and production assistance; and to Mike Sweat, Johannes van Dam, John Stoeckel, Chris Castle, Kristin Banek, and Barbara Janowitz, who reviewed all or part of the *Handbook* and provided many helpful comments.

Population Council
1 Dag Hammarskjold Plaza
New York, NY 10017 USA

4301 Connecticut Avenue NW
Suite 280
Washington, DC 20008 USA
horizons@pcdc.org
www.popcouncil.org

Andrew A. Fisher, ScD, is senior associate at the Population Council and director of the Horizons Program, a global HIV/AIDS operations research project implemented by the Population Council.

James R. Foreit, DrPH, is a senior associate at the Population Council. He works on the Council's FRONTIERS Program, which conducts operations research globally on reproductive health topics.

John Laing, PhD, was a senior associate with the Population Council in South and East Asia. He is currently retired.

John Stoeckel, PhD, formerly a senior associate with the Population Council in South and East Asia, is now a health consultant based in Bangkok, Thailand.

John Townsend, PhD, is director of the Frontiers in Reproductive Health Program of the Population Council.

Contents

PREFACE

The *Handbook* has several objectives and thus several uses. First and foremost, it is designed to help HIV/AIDS researchers develop and write a detailed operations research proposal. An appropriate use of the *Handbook* is as a resource in workshops or courses on research design and proposal development. Thus, the organization of the *Handbook* follows that of a research proposal, starting with identifying, defining, and justifying a research problem, and ending with how to prepare a budget. The chapters in between cover a variety of topics such as research objectives, study design, data tabulation, data analysis, and dissemination and utilization of research findings.

Although the *Handbook* is not an academic textbook on research methods, it does provide a review of many key concepts and important methods essential for conducting HIV/AIDS field research studies. These features can also help HIV/AIDS program administrators and managers as well as health policymakers understand the process of operations research and the uses of research findings to improve HIV/AIDS service delivery.

The *Handbook* assumes that the reader has some familiarity with the terms and concepts of research design and statistics as well as some experience with research studies, particularly those that address issues concerning HIV/AIDS. Most of the examples in the *Handbook* were drawn from actual HIV/AIDS operations research studies conducted in Asia, Africa, and Latin America by the Horizons Program.

Funded by the U.S. Agency for International Development, Horizons is a global HIV/AIDS operations research program implemented by the Population Council in collaboration with the International Center for Research on Women (ICRW), the International HIV/AIDS Alliance, the Program for Appropriate Technology in Health (PATH), Tulane University, Family Health International (FHI), and Johns Hopkins University (JHU).

ACRONYMS AND ABBREVIATIONS

ANOVA	analysis of variance
ARV	antiretroviral
CBO	community-based organization
CDC	Centers for Disease Control and Prevention
CEA	cost-effectiveness analysis
DOTS	Directory Observed Treatment Short Course
FHI	Family Health International
HAART	highly active antiretroviral therapy
ICRW	International Center for Research on Women
IEC	information, education, and communication
ILO	International Labor Organization
IRB	Institutional Review Board
JHU	Johns Hopkins University
MIS	management information system
MTCT	mother-to-child transmission
NGO	nongovernmental organization
NIH	National Institutes of Health
OR	operations research
PATH	Program for Appropriate Technology in Health
PLHA	people living with HIV/AIDS
PSU	primary sampling unit
RA	randomly assigned
SDP	service delivery point
STI	sexually transmitted infection
UCSF	University of California-San Francisco
USAID	U.S. Agency for International Development
VCT	voluntary testing and counseling

CHAPTER 1

INTRODUCTION

What Is Operations Research?

As HIV/AIDS continues to spread and affect the lives of millions of people, a growing sense of urgency has developed about the imperative need to stop the epidemic. In all areas of the world, national HIV/AIDS programs, along with countless nongovernmental organizations (NGOs) and community-based organizations (CBOs), have initiated programs to expand the response to the epidemic. The goal of these efforts is to prevent the transmission of HIV and to mitigate the consequences of AIDS through care, support, and treatment. The programs range from very large national efforts to very small local efforts. Whatever their size, the programs almost always involve some elements of planning, coordination, service delivery, and involvement of communities and people living with HIV/AIDS (PLHA).

All HIV/AIDS service delivery programs face complex tasks. Behavior change strategies typically require managers to use multiple media channels to spread prevention messages to different social groups. The distribution of condoms, antiretrovirals (ARVs), and other medicines depends on complex logistics systems. Training is often required for a variety of personnel, ranging from doctors, nurses, and other clinical staff to health policymakers, program managers, and volunteers working through NGOs at the local level. In order to be effective and sustainable, these and many other aspects of programs need to be implemented in settings where communities are involved and mobilized.

HIV/AIDS programs are complex because the disease is complex. It affects all aspects of human society—from the cultural sphere to the religious, political, and economic spheres. The infected and affected are many in number, diverse in nature, and widely dispersed throughout the world. HIV/AIDS programs usually address such sensitive issues as sexuality and longstanding concerns about human rights, poverty, economic development, gender inequality, stigma, and discrimination. To be effective, HIV/AIDS programs require not only community involvement and dedicated, committed personnel, but also detailed planning at all levels, close coordination of program implementation efforts, careful training and supervision of personnel, and continuous evaluation of program development and impact. Operations research (OR) is a critically important way to support and inform these essential planning, coordinating, training, and evaluation functions.

OR is a process, a way of identifying and solving program problems. As currently applied in many health and development fields, operations research can be defined as a continuous process with five basic steps:

1. Problem identification and diagnosis.
2. Strategy selection.
3. Strategy testing and evaluation.
4. Information dissemination.
5. Information utilization.

The goal of OR is to increase the efficiency, effectiveness, and quality of services delivered by providers, and the availability, accessibility, and acceptability of services desired by users.

The Focus and Objectives of Operations Research

HIV/AIDS operations research focuses on the day-to-day activities or "operations" of HIV/AIDS programs. These operations are under the control of managers and administrators working in the public and private sectors. The operations consist of training, commodity logistics, voluntary counseling and testing, public information and education, hospital and clinic activities, orphan support, community- and home-based care for PLHA, institutional capacity building for NGOs, community mobilization, and many other operations that

are part of HIV/AIDS prevention and mitigation programs. OR looks at problems affecting these service delivery operations, focusing on the search for solutions or, in the language of research, variables that can be manipulated through administrative action.

HIV/AIDS operations research yields answers to perceived program problems. An important objective of OR is to provide managers, administrators, and policymakers with the information they need to improve or scale up existing delivery activities and to plan future ones. OR seeks practical solutions to problem situations and viable alternatives to unsatisfactory operating methods. It diagnoses and evaluates the problems that programs have and compares one service delivery approach against another in terms of impact, cost-effectiveness, quality, and acceptability to clients.

Categories of Operations Research Studies

Operations research studies can be classified under four headings:

Exploratory/Diagnostic Studies: Problem Not Known

These studies seek to determine the parameters of a problem situation before programming begins. In an effort to respond as quickly as possibly to a devastating epidemic, HIV/AIDS programs sometimes were hastily planned and rapidly implemented without a clear understanding of the underlying nature of the problem the program was designed to address. Exploratory/diagnostic studies examine the basic factors influencing a problem situation that need to be addressed later through planned programs.

Exploratory/diagnostic studies are retrospective or cross-sectional in design. This type of study is most often undertaken before a program is implemented whenever there is a perceived problem but the nature of the problem and the correct program responses to it are not known. A key aspect of these studies is the search for programmatically manipulatable variables.

Field Intervention Studies: Program Approach Not Known

These studies test, on an experimental basis, new approaches or solutions to overcoming a program problem. They can be thought of as "proof of concept" studies. In many situations, an earlier exploratory/diagnostic study has identified the factors responsible for a problem, but the most effective and efficient solution for alleviating the problem is not known. Field intervention studies test new HIV/AIDS service delivery approaches. These studies are always prospective and longitudinal and usually employ either an experimental or quasi-experimental research design.

Evaluative Studies: Impact Not Known

Very often, HIV/AIDS activities are implemented for years but never assessed. In such cases, evaluative studies can be a valuable operations research approach for examining retrospectively or cross-sectionally the effect of program activities. Evaluation is an ongoing process that should occur continually over the life of a program.

Cost-effectiveness Studies: Cost and Effectiveness Not Known

In many cases, the overall impact of a program in terms of increasing knowledge about HIV, changing unsafe sex practices, or reducing HIV transmission may be known, but the cost and particularly the cost-effectiveness of the program are unknown. For program managers who have to make difficult decisions about allocating scarce resources, cost-effectiveness studies can be a valuable management tool, and cost-effectiveness analyses are frequently part of intervention and evaluation studies.

These four categories of OR studies are not mutually exclusive. Frequently a single OR study will begin with an exploratory/diagnostic phase to identify key variables of importance. During the second phase, a field intervention might be initiated to test different program solutions to overcoming the problem. Subsequently, an evaluative phase might be implemented to determine the impact of the intervention. Finally, a cost-effectiveness analysis might be undertaken to examine the cost required to obtain a particular unit of effect.

The Methods and Study Designs of Operations Research

The methods of OR range from the qualitative to the quantitative, and the study designs from the non-experimental to the true experimental (see chapter 7). There is no single set of methods or designs unique to operations research. Indeed, it is not the application of a particular set of methods or the use of one design over another that distinguishes OR from other forms of research. Rather, it is the focus or objective of the research.

Simply stated and in its broadest terms, the objective of operations research is to improve the delivery of services. While OR studies may use experimental or non-experimental designs and may include a quantitative analysis of outcome measures or a qualitative consideration of health issues, the central objective always is to obtain a better understanding of the "operations" of programs so that needed improvements can be made.

Illustrative Topics for HIV/AIDS Operations Research Studies

Hundreds of HIV/AIDS studies have been implemented throughout the world. The range of potential topics for HIV/AIDS operations research is vast. Most of these topics fall under two primary categories—**prevention of HIV transmission** or **mitigation of the effects of HIV/AIDS**. These two areas are not mutually exclusive. A few topics fall under both of these categories, such as stigma reduction, discrimination, and other human rights violations that hamper efforts to prevent HIV transmission and to provide care, support, and treatment to those affected by HIV/AIDS.

Prevention of HIV transmission remains a key strategy for reducing the effects of the epidemic on future generations. Most prevention strategies focus on changing sexual behaviors and require a clear understanding of the social context within which the behaviors take place. Mitigation strategies usually consist of care, support, and treatment activities that address the needs of PLHA, orphans, and other vulnerable groups. For the purpose of illustration only, we list below some topic areas that are associated with prevention or mitigation and that are often the focus of operations research studies.

Selected Topic Areas for Operations Research on HIV Prevention

Condom Promotion
Promotion of both male and female condoms continues to receive major attention in most countries. But consistent condom use remains an elusive goal. Many OR studies examine different approaches to obtaining higher and more consistent levels of condom use among groups most vulnerable to sexually transmitted infections (STIs). Programs often use behavior change communications to encourage safe sex practices.

Prevention and Management of STIs
The presence of STIs greatly facilitates the transmission of HIV. Strategies to prevent and control STIs through condom promotion, the use of peer educators, and periodic presumptive treatment with antibiotics have been the focus of several OR studies.

Voluntary Counseling and Testing (VCT)
VCT programs are often the link between prevention and mitigation activities. For those who test negative for HIV, VCT can be a powerful incentive to change high-risk sexual or injecting drug use behavior in order to remain negative. For those who test positive, VCT can serve as a link to care, support, and treatment options. In many countries, OR has tested new approaches to encourage people to seek VCT.

Reaching Young People
Youth, particularly young girls, are highly vulnerable to HIV infection. OR studies that address youth issues sometimes focus on school-based youth or out-of-school youth. Most programs seek to increase access to information and services for youth, sometimes by using peer educators. A particularly important role for OR is testing new programmatic approaches that address gender and power issues within sexual relations and that seek to increase the self-esteem of girls.

Prevention of Mother-to-Child Transmission (MTCT)
Numerous MTCT issues can be addressed through OR. Examples include exploring different ways to involve men more actively in the counseling and care of pregnant women, testing strategies for mobilizing communities to support MTCT programs, and testing counselor training strategies.

MAINTAINING PREVENTIVE BEHAVIORS

Preventing HIV transmission requires sustained safe sex behaviors for a lifetime. A major challenge for programs is how to find effective ways to sustain these behaviors for extended periods.

INTEGRATING FAMILY PLANNING AND HIV/AIDS SERVICES

Family planning programs present an opportunity to introduce HIV/AIDS education and services, and HIV/AIDS programs provide a similar opportunity to introduce family planning services. OR studies have been directed at promoting condoms for dual protection, which means protection against both pregnancy and STIs, including HIV. A major challenge for OR is to develop and test cost-effective strategies for integrating these services.

Selected Topic Areas for Operations Research on AIDS Mitigation

ASSISTING ORPHANS

Large increases in adult mortality due to AIDS have been followed by large increases in AIDS orphans. The death of one or both parents affects orphans in many ways, causing setbacks in education, health, nutrition, and psychosocial wellbeing, as well as increased vulnerability to HIV and STI infection. OR studies are urgently needed to identify cost-effective models for assisting AIDS orphans.

ADMINISTERING ANTIRETROVIRAL THERAPY

With the decrease in the cost of antiretroviral (ARV) drugs, many countries and organizations within countries are initiating treatment programs for PLHA. These programs face numerous operational issues that urgently need to be addressed. For example, what is the best way to ensure that a logistics system provides an uninterrupted supply of drugs? How can high levels of adherence to ARVs be maintained among patients? What is the role of community-based organizations in ARV programs? When should ARVs be administered? Can nonphysicians administer ARVs safely and with high standards of quality of care? These and many other issues concerning ARVs can be addressed through operations research.

BUILDING THE CAPACITY OF PLHA ORGANIZATIONS

In most countries of the world, PLHA support groups have been formed. OR is needed to find ways of strengthening and sustaining the capacity of these groups by, for example, providing ongoing psychosocial support to PLHA as they deal with fear, guilt, stigma, anger, depression, discrimination, and isolation from society.

IMPACT ON FAMILY CAREGIVERS

HIV/AIDS has had a huge impact on family caregivers. Caregivers often suffer from grief, exhaustion, isolation, and a lack of resources to help family members suffering from AIDS. OR studies need to test ways of reaching family caregivers to alleviate these problems.

Expanded Example of Operations Research Topics Related to Access to Treatment

The complexity of HIV/AIDS and the numerous topics that could be addressed through operations research is best illustrated by presenting an expanded example of the topics concerning just one area: access to treatment with antiretrovirals and to treatment of opportunistic infections. Little is known about the many operational issues that face countries trying to initiate large-scale drug treatment programs using ARVs and other drugs. A research question of significant importance is how to ensure the safe and effective administration of drugs on a continuous and uninterrupted basis to the largest number of infected people at the lowest possible cost. Some of the many questions about expanding access to treatment that could be addressed through OR studies are listed below.

SERVICE DELIVERY

Policymakers and program managers dealing with treatment issues face many unknowns. For example, most health care workers in the world, including physicians and nurses, have received very little if any training in the delivery of ARVs. What kind of training do these health care workers need to develop the competence to deliver ARVs, and how long should that training last? The delivery of ARVs also requires substantial attention to a host of health services, administration, and infrastructure issues, including supplies, equipment, record keeping, and expanded VCT services. The health care systems of most developing countries are already severely constrained and have difficulty delivering even the most basic curative drugs. Can these systems be rapidly upgraded to deliver far more complex ARVs? OR studies that address this question need to be implemented.

BEHAVIOR

OR also needs to examine better ways to improve patient adherence to complex drug regimens. Antiretrovirals must often be taken at fixed times of the day and in particular combinations for a lifetime. Frequently, patients experience side effects that can discourage continued use of the drugs. What is the best way to ensure patient adherence? One suggestion is to adapt a Directly Observed Treatment Short Course (DOTS) approach similar to that used to treat tuberculosis. The tuberculosis DOTS program, however, is not always successful, and with HIV/ AIDS there is the added complication that every day patients must identify themselves as infected and thus risk stigma, discrimination, and possibly violence. How can high levels of adherence to drug regimens be maintained to get the maximum benefit from the drugs and avoid the development of resistant HIV strains that can occur when adherence is low?

EQUITY

ARV treatments are not likely to be available in sufficient quantities for everyone who needs them, a situation that raises human rights, ethical, and gender issues about who gets treatment. Which policies and procedures can best ensure equitable and nondiscriminatory access to ARVs and other drugs? What role does gender play in obtaining access to drugs?

COMMUNITY MOBILIZATION

While it is clear that the public health care system in many countries will not be able to meet all treatment needs, it is not yet clear which other institutions and organizations could become involved. OR can help NGOs and community-based organizations effectively mobilize to play a supportive role in treatment.

PRIVATE SECTOR

The private sector is likely to be a major actor in the delivery of ARVs. Increasingly, many companies and other private sector groups in some countries have indicated that they will begin to provide ARVs to their workforce. However, the best ways to provide these drugs while maintaining the confidentiality of workers is not known.

COST

Cost issues will be crucial in the delivery of ARVs. Which program approaches can be used to keep costs low? Besides the costs of drugs, what are other program costs involved in increasing access to drugs, and how can these costs be reduced to a minimum?

These are just a few of the many research questions about access to treatment. Other HIV/AIDS topics such as mother-to-child transmission, voluntary counseling and testing, stigma, and discrimination are equally complex and raise numerous questions that can be answered through operations research.

CHAPTER 2

IDENTIFYING, DEFINING, AND JUSTIFYING THE RESEARCH PROBLEM

Problem Identification

The proposal-writing process always begins with a statement of a problem. Countless problems face HIV/AIDS programs. Finding a problem therefore is not difficult, but identifying one for the purpose of research is not always easy.

One of the most important first tasks of research is to identify and define clearly the problem you wish to study. If you are uncertain about the research problem or if you are not clear in your own mind about what you want to study, others who read your proposal will also be uncertain. A well-defined research problem statement leads naturally to the statement of research objectives, to the hypotheses, to a definition of key variables, and to a selection of a methodology for measuring the variables. A poorly defined research problem leads to confusion.

All research is set in motion by the existence of a problem. A problem is a perceived difficulty, a feeling of discomfort about the way things are, or a discrepancy between what someone believes should be the situation and what is in reality the situation. While problems are the initiating force behind research, not all problems require research. A potential research situation arises when three conditions exist:

1. A perceived discrepancy exists between what is and what should be.
2. A question exists about why there is a discrepancy.
3. At least two possible and plausible answers exist to the question.

The last point is important. If there is only one possible and plausible answer to the question about the discrepancy, then a research situation does not exist.

Example of a Nonresearch Problem

PROBLEM SITUATION
A recent situation analysis assessment of a hospital in District A found that 125 HIV-positive adults were coming to the hospital every day as part of a DOTS program to take medication for tuberculosis (TB). But last month's service statistics from the hospital's DOTS program revealed that for one entire week, none of the 125 patients received any medication.

DISCREPANCY
All 125 patients should be receiving a daily treatment for TB, but all 125 did not receive a single treatment for an entire week last month.

PROBLEM QUESTION
What factor or factors are responsible for 125 patients' failing to receive any treatment for their TB for an entire week?

ANSWER
During the week when the patients didn't receive daily TB treatments, a very heavy rainstorm caused flooding that washed out several roads and destroyed a major bridge that is used to bring supplies to the district hospital. Because of the flooding and the destroyed bridge, the hospital ran out of TB medication, and a resupply truck could not reach the hospital for one week while the bridge was being repaired.

In this example, a problem situation exists, but the reason for the problem is already known. Therefore, assuming that all the facts are correct, there is no reason to conduct research on the factors associated with the break in the supply of daily TB medication for 125 patients. Nonetheless, there may very well be a need to conduct research on the question of why the supply logistics system is incapable of providing medication during the rainy season, when it is known that roads and bridges are frequently damaged.

Example of a Research Problem

PROBLEM SITUATION
District A almost always experiences flooding during the rainy season. Recognizing this problem, the National HIV/AIDS Program, working with the Ministry of Health, established a new supply logistics system for the district. Just before the rainy season, each hospital and health post in the district is given a four-month supply of medication to cover TB and other AIDS-related opportunistic infections. In addition, the Ministry of Health maintains several small motorboats in the district that can be used to transport supplies across rivers where there is either no bridge or the bridge has been destroyed. Despite these new measures, this

year's service statistics from District A indicate that a large number of PLHA enrolled in the DOTS program failed to receive daily medication for TB.

DISCREPANCY
The new supply logistics system should be able to ensure a continuous supply of medication during the rainy season, but this year large numbers of TB patients did not receive medication during much of the rainy season.

PROBLEM QUESTION
Why has the new supply logistics system been incapable of delivering needed medication to HIV-positive TB patients?

POSSIBLE ANSWERS
- An order for new medical supplies was not placed in time before the beginning of the rainy season.
- The motorboats used to transport supplies in emergencies were not working.
- Because of severe flooding, many patients could not reach the DOTS service delivery points on a daily basis.

In this example, there are several possible and plausible reasons for the problem situation. One or more of these reasons might be correct, and at least two of the possible problems may be under the control of managers to fix: ordering drugs on time and improving maintenance of the boats. Therefore, this is a potential research situation.

In some situations, it is relatively easy to identify the problem, define it, hypothesize the reasons for it, and conduct operations research to determine which reason is correct or more nearly correct. The reasons for the supply logistics problem in the example above could probably be determined fairly easily and certainly would not require an extended and expensive research study. Other problems, such as the one in the next example, are not so easy to identify or study.

Example of a Research Problem

PROBLEM SITUATION
A recent provincial study revealed great differences among villages in the prevalence of HIV-positive persons. Despite the fact that all villages receive the same level of health education and services from the Ministry of Health, some villages have an HIV prevalence rate as high as 32 percent among adults from 15 to 49 years old, while other villages have a rate as low as 6 percent.

DISCREPANCY
In a relatively small geographic area, you would expect that all villages should have approximately the same seroprevalence rate but, in fact, there is great variation among villages.

PROBLEM QUESTION
Which factors are responsible for the geographic variation in HIV prevalence among villages?

POSSIBLE ANSWERS
- Villages differ in their socioeconomic environments, and these differences influence the context within which HIV is transmitted. Some are stable agricultural villages, while some are mobile fishing communities. Some villages are located on major roads and have easy access to market towns; others are more remote with very difficult access to market centers. Some villages have schools, health clinics, electricity, and a good water supply, while others do not have these advantages. These and many other social, economic, and cultural differences affect the context within which sexual relations take place and HIV is transmitted.
- Villages differ in individual and institutional support for HIV/AIDS prevention, care, and support programs. In some villages, influential local leaders strongly support sexual behavior change and condom distribution programs. In other villages, people are resistant to these

programs, and there is substantial stigma and discrimination associated with HIV/AIDS. In some villages, there are very active anti-AIDS clubs for youth, strong PLHA organizations, and effective orphan care NGOs. In other villages these institutions are absent. These differences in individual commitment to and institutional support for HIV/AIDS programs affect the sexual behavior of individuals, the use of condoms, the level of stigma and discrimination, and the transmission of HIV.

While the problem situation presented above is fairly clear, the possible and plausible reasons for the problem are complex. Several of these reasons have been described, but it is very likely there are many more.

In situations such as this one, the researcher must devote considerable time and attention to identifying and clearly defining the problem situation before any potential solutions to the problem can be tested experimentally through a longitudinal operations research study. The aim of clearly identifying and defining a problem situation is to focus the research on the most important aspects of a problem that can be changed through a program intervention. Consider the next example, which also suggests a number of possible reasons for the problem situation.

Example of a Research Problem

Problem Situation

In country A, the National AIDS Program has initiated an experimental project to provide highly active antiretroviral therapy (HAART) drugs to 1,000 persons with AIDS. All of the patients in the program receive extensive individual counseling from trained counselors. They also receive information packets on how and when to take the various pills they receive; these emphasize the need to take the pills exactly as prescribed and describe the possible side effects of the pills. All patients are monitored regularly at a clinic for CD4 cell counts and viral load levels. They are also visited in their homes monthly by trained care providers who answer questions and monitor adherence to the drug regime. Despite these efforts, a recent detailed assessment of all the HAART patients found that 43 percent of them had taken their pills incorrectly over the past month, viral load levels had risen in these patients, and CD4 cells had declined.

Discrepancy

The National AIDS Program prides itself on providing high-quality services to the 1,000 patients with HIV/AIDS in the experimental program. Laboratory equipment is functioning well, drug supplies are available, the lab technicians are trained, the counselors are also trained and supervised, and the information packets given to each patient are comprehensive. Given these conditions, all patients should know how to correctly take their HAART medication, but at least 43 percent of them are not taking the medication correctly.

Problem Question

What factor or factors are responsible for a relatively high level of nonadherence to the drug regime among patients who are counseled and monitored closely?

Possible Answers

- The counselors are inadequately trained to explain in simple terms the complex treatment regime required for patients on antiretrovirals and the consequences of failing to adhere to this regime.
- The information packets received by the patients are too complex, particularly for a population with a low level of literacy, and therefore are not read by many patients.

- The monthly home visits by the care providers had the unexpected effect of identifying patients as HIV-positive to their family and neighbors. Among some patients, this resulted in discrimination and domestic violence, which in turn resulted in patients' discontinuing the medication and requesting that the care providers discontinue the monthly home visits for fear of further discrimination and violence.
- Many patients experienced serious drug side effects, including drug toxicity and drug intolerance, which led to difficulties with adherence to the regime and, in some cases, to nonadherence.
- In some patients, the HAART regime was highly effective, and the patients gained weight and a sense of health that they had not experienced in a long time. Unfortunately, one unexpected consequence of this was that some patients decided they no longer needed the HAART and stopped taking their medication.

In this example, the problem situation is clear: A survey of HIV-positive persons found that 43 percent did not adhere to a prescribed antiretroviral drug regime. A discrepancy exists: With the availability of counseling, information packets, and home visits, HIV-positive patients should know how to take their drugs correctly, but 43 percent do not take their drugs correctly.

The discrepancy between what should be and what is suggests a problem question and five possible answers to the question. It is not known which of these five possible answers are correct or more nearly correct. All possible and plausible answers could relate to factors under the control of program managers. This is a situation that requires research.

Problem Definition

Identifying a problem situation is the first essential step in designing a research proposal, but it must then be followed by a process of problem definition. The research problem identified must now be defined in terms of its occurrence, intensity, distribution, and other measures for which data are already available. The aim is to determine all that is currently known about the problem and the reason it exists.

While it is always possible to guess why a problem exists, guesses are often wrong and usually do not provide a firm basis for designing a research study. A far better way to define a problem situation is to review relevant literature, examine current service statistics, seek educated opinions from persons concerned about the problem, and obtain probable reasons for the problem from social, economic, or health theory. A careful social, economic, and epidemiologic diagnosis of problems related to HIV and AIDS should always be made. In other words, how widespread is the problem? Who is affected by the problem? What is its distribution? How often does the problem occur? What social or cultural practices are associated with the problem? What costs are associated with the problem? A good social, economic, and epidemiologic diagnosis will help establish the parameters of the problem and help the research investigator and program managers determine the following:

Incidence and Prevalence

Incidence is the number of new cases (people) who get a disease such as HIV during a specific period of time. Prevalence is the total number of people who have the disease at a specific point in time. Often, people talk about an incidence rate, which is the number of new cases of a disease that occur during a specific time period divided by the total number of people exposed to the risk of developing the disease during that same period. Similarly, the prevalence rate is the total number of people with the disease at a specific time divided by the total number of people in the population at that time.

Geographic Areas Affected

It is important to know whether particular geographic regions are affected by the problem. Does the problem generally occur only in rural areas? Does it also affect those who live in cities? Is the problem restricted to mountain areas, coastal areas, or island areas?

Characteristics of Population Groups Affected

Are there special population groups affected by the problem, such as young girls, miners, truckers, sex workers, newborn infants, men who have sex with men, and injecting drug users?

Probable Reasons for the Problem

A review of information on a problem should suggest a number of probable reasons why the problem exists. What is the current thinking about the reasons for the problem? Is there general agreement among many people about the reasons, or are there many different, conflicting views?

Possible Solutions

Many projects and programs may have been directed at the problem in an attempt to overcome it. What types of solutions have been tried in the past? How successful have past efforts been? Have lessons already been learned about how to address the problem? What approaches to solving the problem seem to work? What approaches seem not to work?

Unanswered Questions

From the review of information on the problem, what seem to be the unanswered questions about it? What aspects of the problem need to be further researched?

Reviewing what is already known about a problem is an essential part of the research process. A good review of information will suggest the social, economic, political, and health importance of the problem. It will help to narrow the focus of the proposed research and will indicate major theoretical concepts and operational variables other researchers have considered important. It will suggest possible research hypotheses that need to be tested. Finally, it will prevent the investigator from reinventing the wheel or, in other words, conducting research on a problem that has already been researched many times in the past with fairly consistent findings.

Example of a Research Problem Identification and Definition Statement

In Zambia, a pilot program was initiated to train volunteers to provide home-based care for PLHA. The expectation was that this program would provide a more cost-effective means of assisting PLHA than using full-time paid nurses. The volunteers were trained for three weeks. They visited the homes of PLHA once a week to provide palliative care, social and psychological support, basic information about HIV/AIDS, and referral to the closest health center.

A unique aspect of the program was the development of a simple algorithm that the caregivers could use to help diagnose the various conditions the PLHA complained about, such as diarrhea, rashes, fever, cough, and headaches. Depending on the nature of the condition diagnosed, the caregiver would either provide simple medicines such as aspirin or refer the person to the nearest medical center. The program was expected to serve as a cost-effective model, particularly in rural areas, where there are large numbers of PLHA but relatively few health care facilities and virtually no outreach programs using more highly trained personnel such as nurses.

Although some of the volunteers were quite active in making regular home visits to PLHA, many of the volunteers were not as active or committed. Indeed, over time, more and more of the volunteers either dropped out of the program or significantly decreased the amount of time they devoted to caring for PLHA and making home visits. A diagnostic study of the volunteer program indicated several difficulties:

- While the involvement of volunteers to make home visits is obviously less costly than using full-time paid nurses, it is not necessarily as effective. Volunteers may or may not have the time or motivation to visit homes regularly. Typically, the initial motivation and enthusiasm quickly wanes and after a period of some months the volunteers visit few, if any, homes.
- Working with HIV/AIDS-affected people is not easy, even for the most dedicated volunteers. Many of the volunteers developed strong emotional ties with the PLHA they visited. The death of a PLHA was emotionally stressful for the volunteer and often led to a sense of despair, followed by an inability to continue as a home-based caregiver.
- The area assigned to each volunteer, usually several villages, was too large for one person to cover adequately. The volunteers tended to use an ad hoc method for making home visits and did not have a coordinated, scheduled plan. One result of this was that the volunteers visited some houses far more often than others.
- There was little or no supervision of the volunteers in the field. This may be one reason that the enthusiasm of many volunteers declines. While PLHA need social and psychological support, caregivers also need the same type of support from supervisors.

- Although the volunteers completed an initial three-week training course, no effort was made to provide them with ongoing training that might have served to strengthen and reinforce their skills.
- Reports from PLHA who had been visited by the volunteers suggested that the information provided during home visits was superficial and not very helpful. Many volunteers apparently were unable to give the type of specific information about opportunistic infections that the PLHA desired. Also, PLHA stated that the volunteers were simply not able to alleviate most of the problems they had.

The findings from the diagnostic study were discussed extensively by the project management team and the district health authorities. It is not known which one of these problems or which combination of them is affecting the volunteer home-based care program the most. On the basis of the diagnostic study, several possible solutions to the problems have been proposed:

- It might be possible to eliminate the volunteers entirely and replace them with full-time paid nurses. These nurses would undoubtedly devote more time to home visits and would probably provide more detailed information and a greater range of services to the PLHA. However, using nurses might result in an extremely costly home care program that probably would not be sustainable in the long run. Moreover, relatively few nurses are available for this kind of work.
- A second alternative might be to retrain the volunteers. While this solution would cost less than having full-time paid nurses provide home-based care, it is not likely to solve all of the problems. The area assigned to each volunteer would still be too large to be covered effectively. There would still be a need to establish an effective supervisory system. Follow-up of clients might still be a problem, and even though the knowledge and skills of

the volunteers might improve, there would still be the problem of emotional burnout resulting in volunteers dropping out from the program.

- A third alternative might be to combine the first two suggestions. Volunteers could be retrained, and a regular program of supervision by nurses could be instituted. On a selective basis, the nurses could make home visits to PLHA most in need of more comprehensive medical services. The geographical area covered by the volunteers could be reduced. An improved referral system with the health posts could be established. Finally, regular refresher training could help the volunteers deal with the emotional distress of working with PLHA.

Comments on the Example

The first paragraph focuses on just one country, Zambia, and on just one home-based care program for PLHA. It was expected that the use of volunteers would be a cost-effective alternative to using full-time paid nurses.

The second paragraph notes a problem situation, a discrepancy between what was expected and what actually happened. It was expected that the volunteers would be an effective alternative to nurses. What happened, however, was that the volunteers began to drop out of the program or significantly reduced the amount of time they devoted to caring for PLHA. A diagnostic study of the volunteer program suggested six possible problem areas.

The third paragraph notes that the problems identified by the diagnostic study have been extensively discussed by the project management team and the district health authorities. Several possible solutions for overcoming the problems were presented. The first two were rejected as being inadequate for one reason or another. The third solution, a combination of the first two solutions, was accepted as the most likely to succeed and thus is the solution to be tested in an operations research intervention study.

What To Do: Problem Identification and Definition

1. Follow this general procedure when identifying and defining a problem situation:

   - Start with a simple statement of the problem situation.
   - Add details as you review the literature, review theoretical concepts, and investigate the problem in greater depth.
   - Simplify the focus by identifying the most important aspects of the problem that are researchable.

2. Make a first attempt at identifying the problem situation by using the following format:

   - Problem Situation: Write a small, simple paragraph that identifies the problem.
   - Discrepancy: State the discrepancy between what is and what should be.
   - Problem Question: Write down the central problem question.
   - Possible Answers: Write two or more plausible answers to the problem question.

3. From available research literature, health and behavioral theory, current service statistics, educated opinions, the assistance of PLHA, and other sources of information, try to add details to the problem situation you have just identified. Look for theoretical concepts and operational variables that you may have missed. List these concepts and variables on a piece of paper as you come across them. Try to answer the following questions:

   - What are the incidence and prevalence of the problem?
   - Which geographic areas are affected by the problem?
   - Which population groups are affected by the problem?
   - What are the findings of other research studies?
   - What has been done to overcome the problem in the past?
   - How successful were past efforts to overcome the problem?
   - What seem to be major unanswered questions about the problem?

4. With the information you have collected from a literature review and other sources, rewrite your statement identifying and defining the problem. Use the format described above: Problem Situation, Discrepancy, Problem Question, and Possible Answers. Add details that help to define the problem, but organize the information. Try to establish the boundaries of the problem. Focus your attention on the most important, researchable aspects of the problem.

5. Have one or more colleagues read your final statement identifying and defining the problem situation. Have them tell you what he or she thinks the problem is. If they are unclear about the problem situation or cannot describe the discrepancy between what is and what should be, then go back to the beginning and start all over again.

Problem Justification

Now that you have identified and defined the problem situation, it is necessary next to justify the importance of the problem. Research often is expensive and time consuming. Ask yourself why the problem you wish to study is important. Can you justify your selection of the research problem? Can you convince others that the problem is important?

Example for Justifying the Selection of a Research Problem

Over time, millions of HIV-infected people in Africa and elsewhere in the world are developing HIV-related illnesses. In most African countries, hospitals, clinics, and other formal health care system institutions simply cannot cope with the large numbers of people in need of physical care and social and psychological support. In some hospitals, well over half of the beds are already occupied by AIDS patients; in some countries the figure is as high as 70 percent of all hospital beds. This is a problem of great concern to health care planners, as well as to the Ministry of Finance, which simply does not have the resources to build new facilities or train large numbers of new providers.

The problem of providing care and support for PLHA is particularly challenging in rural areas because there are relatively few health facilities or adequately trained providers available. In this situation, an alternative is to provide care, support, and treatment in the homes of those with AIDS. How to do this in a cost-effective manner while simultaneously providing high-quality services is a challenge. New models of delivering care and support services in rural areas need to be developed and tested to improve the quality of life for PLHA. Without effective new approaches, large numbers of people with AIDS will suffer physical and psychological pain that might otherwise be avoided or at least lessened.

Comments on the Example

The first paragraph establishes the dimensions of the problem. The large number of people with AIDS cannot be adequately treated or supported by the formal health care system, which is already overwhelmed in many countries. The second paragraph notes that the problem is particularly acute in rural areas, where health facilities and providers are relatively few in number. An alternative is to provide services to PLHA in their homes. The important question is how to do this. The paragraph ends by saying that without the development of new approaches to care and support, large numbers of PLHA will needlessly suffer.

What To Do: Justifying the Selection of a Research Problem

1. In justifying the importance of a research problem, it is helpful to ask yourself a series of questions and then try to answer each of them.

   - Is the problem you wish to study a current and timely one? Does the problem exist now?
   - How widespread is the problem? Are many areas and many people affected by the problem?
   - Does the problem affect key populations, such as youth, PLHA, mothers, or children?
   - Does the problem relate to ongoing program activities?
   - Does the problem relate to broad social, economic, and health issues, such as unemployment, income distribution, poverty, the status of women, or education?
   - Who else is concerned about the problem? Are top government officials concerned? Are medical doctors or other professionals concerned?

2. Review your answers to these questions, and arrange them into one or two paragraphs that justify the importance of the research problem. Start by discussing the broad issues that justify the problem and then begin to focus on the more specific issues related to a particular population group or geographical setting.

Involving Program Managers and Others in the Research Process

One important way to accomplish the first step in the OR process is to involve not only researchers but also program managers and many other people, such as village chiefs, teachers, health personnel, NGOs, and PLHA organizations, in the entire problem identification, definition, and justification process. This involvement links the program experience of managers with the HIV/AIDS problem experience and understanding of PLHA with the technical and methodological skills of researchers.

Teaming researchers, program managers, and PLHA is an educational experience for everyone that can have long-range benefits that go far beyond the mere design and implementation of a single OR study. Researchers, for example, begin to understand more fully the day-to-day administrative concerns of managers, the service delivery problems NGOs face, and the social, economic, psychological, and health concerns that PLHA confront every day. This increased understanding can help sharpen the focus of a study on those aspects of a program problem that could be changed.

Administrators begin to appreciate the need to identify and define program problems on the basis of accurate data. They begin to view research as an important tool for decision making and as an ongoing process to which they can contribute.

PLHA begin to experience a sense of empowerment and hope for the future as they become involved in identifying problem situations that affect their lives but could be changed through an operations research process. The early involvement of all key stakeholders in the operations research process is more likely to increase their interest later in reviewing and using the results from OR studies.

CHAPTER 3

STRATEGY SELECTION TO SOLVE THE PROBLEM

Examples of Strategies to Test

After having identified, defined, and justified a research problem, the next step in the operations research process is to select a strategy that can be tested to overcome the problem. Just as countless problems affect HIV/AIDS programs, an equal number of potential solutions to these problems exist. A few examples of strategies that have been tested through OR interventions in Asia, Latin America, and Africa are listed below:

Integrating HIV/AIDS services into a family planning program by focusing on condoms as a means of providing dual protection from pregnancy and HIV and other STIs, and of achieving greater male involvement in family planning.

Implementing a 100 percent condom use policy in brothels by working with brothel owners, training sex workers in negotiation skills, and introducing the female condom in addition to the male condom.

Working with private sector companies to develop and implement nondiscriminatory and nonstigmatizing HIV/AIDS policies in the workplace.

Developing and implementing life skills education courses for school-based youth by training teachers and youth peer educators.

Reducing STIs among sex workers and miners through peer educators, condom promotion, and periodic presumptive treatment for STIs.

Reducing mother-to-child transmission of HIV through voluntary counseling and testing of pregnant women, antiretroviral treatment with AZT or nevirapine, and breast milk substitutes for those who test positive.

Building the capacity of NGOs through a process of self-diagnosis of organizational problem areas and greater involvement of PLHA in planning and service delivery.

Helping children who will soon become orphans by working with their AIDS-affected parents before they die to appoint a guardian, settle issues of property to avoid land grabbing by relatives after death, and linking the children with community support groups that can help with school fees.

Developing new policies and training programs for all levels of hospital staff to create a more friendly and nondiscriminatory environment for PLHA.

Increasing adherence by PLHA to antiretroviral drugs by instituting a directly observed treatment program and by implementing weekly home visits by a nurse.

Assisting men who have sex with men by creating support groups and developing nondiscriminatory health care services.

Reducing violence against women who test positive by involving their partners in voluntary counseling and testing programs.

Guidelines for Selecting an Appropriate Strategy to Test

Before selecting a management or service delivery strategy to test in an operations research study, first go back and review the details of the program problem that concerns you. The nature of the problem should determine the selection of a strategy to test for overcoming the problem. In other words, let the problem determine the selection of the strategy. Don't make the mistake of selecting a strategy solution first and then searching for a problem to which to apply the solution. This may sound like a rather obvious point, but it is surprising how often a single strategy such as social marketing of condoms or the use of more information, education, and communication (IEC) materials (posters, videos, brochures, and pamphlets) is viewed as a panacea and repeatedly applied to almost any program problem whether or not it is the most appropriate strategy.

In addition to carefully reviewing the program problem, there are other guidelines you can follow to help select and develop an appropriate strategy to test in an operations research study.

Review the theories and strategies other people have used to solve similar program problems. One way to do this is to examine the operations research findings from the many HIV/AIDS studies conducted in the past. Find out which management and service delivery strategies seem to work best for particular program problems. What does behavioral or health theory indicate are possible strategies to overcoming the problem? Hold a meeting with the people who are most affected by the problem or most concerned with it. People who are affected by management and service delivery problems (such as PLHA, caregivers, and administrators) usually have opinions, often strong ones, about possible solution strategies that can be used to overcome the problem. It is always important to obtain their ideas since they often can come up with better strategies than anyone else.

Look for strategies that can be implemented without overburdening the implementing institution. If the resource requirements for testing a solution strategy are much greater than the expected benefits, the strategy should be seriously questioned before it is implemented.

Seek strategies that are simple to implement. In deciding between alternative strategies of service delivery with potentially equal impacts, select the strategy that is the simplest in terms of facilities and equipment needed, personnel and training required, time and money spent, logistics and management required, and other considerations. On the other hand, don't sacrifice what might be effective strategies that may be more complex to implement for simple strategies that are not effective.

Develop strategies where the proposed solution is under the control of program managers and acceptable to the community and key stakeholders. A solution strategy, or in the language of research, "the independent variables," must be under the control of the HIV/AIDS program managers. The solution should also be acceptable to the community.

Avoid strategies that are not consistent with the implementing institution's goals, objectives, and development plans. A strategy that does not fall within the current goals, objectives, and plans of an implementing agency may meet with considerable resistance and not receive the resources and attention required for successful implementation.

Select strategies that can be sustained over time. Even if a particular strategy is effective in the short run, that is, during the intervention phase of an operations research study, it is not likely to have much effect on overcoming a program problem if it cannot be sustained by an organization after the OR study is completed. Always seek strategies that have a high probability of being financially sustainable.

Example of a Strategy to Solve the Problem

Approximately 40 percent of HIV/AIDS patients who go to a hospital in Brazil have difficulty taking antiretroviral medication correctly. This is a problem that has many dimensions. Previous research on patient adherence found that poor adherence usually occurs because patients are either not receiving adequate information, are not receiving counseling support to use the information they do receive, or are experiencing severe side effects that are not adequately addressed by providers.

These findings suggest several strategies for reducing adherence problems. First, information materials such as brochures, pamphlets, and a video could be developed and given to all new ARV patients to explain the need for strict adherence to ARV regimens. Second, more intensive one-on-one counseling of new patients could be instituted and followed by monthly group counseling of all ARV patients at clinic settings. Third, a program of monthly home visits by nurses to PLHA could be instituted to provide greater support and to assist patients with the side effects of medication.

Since each of these strategies tends to be complex and each increases program costs, the strategies will be tested sequentially over an 18-month period. First, new IEC materials will be developed and used in the hospital for the first six months. Second, in the next six-month period, more intensive one-on-one and group counseling of ARV patients will be initiated. This second intervention will be added to the first. Finally, in the third six-month period, nurses will make regular monthly visits to the homes of patients who are taking ARVs. This intervention will be added to the two earlier interventions.

Comments on the Example

In this example, previous research has shown that the problem of patients incorrectly taking their antiretroviral medication or failing to take the medication altogether is usually the result of one or more of three factors:

- The patients have not received adequate information.
- They have received the information but have not received adequate counseling to use the information.
- They are experiencing severe side effects without receiving the proper medical attention to overcome the side effects.

Three possible interventions are identified for overcoming the problem. Since these interventions range from the relatively simple (use of information materials for the patients) to the relatively complex and expensive (using nurses for home visits to PLHA), the decision was made to test the interventions sequentially, starting with the simple and then adding on the more complex and expensive interventions.

What To Do: Selecting a Strategy to Test

After a significant program research problem has been identified, defined, and justified, you need to select an appropriate strategy to solve the problem. First, refer to the guidelines for selecting a strategy, including the use of relevant theory, and then in your research proposal:

1. Identify potential strategies that could be used to solve the program problem.

2. Clearly indicate which of the potential strategies you have selected as the most appropriate to solve the program problem.

3. Justify your selection of one or more potential strategies by indicating:

   - Past success with applying the strategy to similar problem situations.
   - The simplicity of implementing the strategy compared to other strategies that are likely to produce the same effect.
   - The potential for sustaining the strategy once the operations research study is completed.

CHAPTER 4

OBJECTIVES AND HYPOTHESES

The objectives and hypotheses of a research study should flow logically from the earlier sections identifying the problem situation, defining the parameters of the problem, and justifying its importance. In this section, we explain how to narrow and focus the research. Specific objectives are written that describe the expected results arising from the study and the outcome variables that will be measured. Once objectives have been set, researchers can formulate specific, testable hypotheses that specify the relationship between program interventions and outcomes.

Ultimate Objectives

Most research studies include a statement of ultimate objectives that describes the expected implications or contributions arising from the study. The ultimate objective of many HIV/AIDS studies is to prevent the transmission of HIV and/or mitigate the impact of AIDS. This is an ambitious goal. It is unlikely that any single study will have a significant effect on reducing HIV transmission or a major effect on mitigating the impact of AIDS. A somewhat more reasonable ultimate objective is that the study will provide program administrators and policymakers with information useful for improving HIV/AIDS programs, scaling up these programs, or developing more effective policies.

Ultimate objectives relate the reasonable and expected contributions of the study to broad social, economic, or health concerns. In this way, the ultimate objectives contribute to the justification of why research on the problem is required. Note, however, that ultimate objectives are **expected contributions**. In a sense, they represent wishful thinking. The investigator does not promise that the contributions will occur and therefore usually does not try to measure them.

Examples of Ultimate Objectives

- "The ultimate objective of this intervention study is to contribute toward improving the quality of life for PLHA and the quality and effectiveness of prevention, care, and support activities offered by community-based organizations to PLHA."
- "The ultimate objective of this intervention study is to develop a cost-effective model of service delivery in Kenya that can reduce the transmission of HIV from mothers to their newborn children."
- "The ultimate objective of this study is to develop for Uganda a cost-effective and sustainable approach for integrating high-quality VCT services with related family planning and STD and TB prevention and care services in primary health care facilities."
- "The ultimate objective of this intervention study is to reduce the transmission of HIV and other STIs by implementing a 100 percent condom use policy in brothels throughout the Dominican Republic."
- "The ultimate objective of this intervention study is to promote in Cambodia the concept of dual protection against STIs and pregnancy through the use of male and female condoms."

Comments on the Examples

Each of these ultimate objectives briefly states the overall expected outcome of the study. These objectives tend to be broad in nature. They represent the expected impact the researchers hope the study will have. Ultimate objectives relate the purpose of the study to larger health concerns, such as improving the quality of life for PLHA, reducing the rate of mother-to-child transmission (MTCT), or integrating HIV/AIDS services with other health care services.

Immediate Objectives

In contrast to ultimate objectives that state what is expected to happen, immediate objectives state what will happen. Immediate objectives relate directly to the research problem situation. They indicate the variables that will be examined and measured. An immediate objective represents a promise by the investigator that certain activities will take place and specific variables will be examined.

Whenever possible, the immediate objective should be stated in **behavioral** terms—in other words, in terms of what actions or behaviors will take place. The immediate objective should specify **who will do, how much of what, to whom, when, where,** and **for what purpose.**

Examples of Immediate Objectives

- "Over a 24-month period, the National HIV/AIDS Prevention Council in Uganda, together with Makerere University, will develop a youth-friendly program to provide comprehensive voluntary counseling and testing six days of every week to youth ages 14 through 24. This program will be evaluated in terms of the number of youth who use the service, the cost-effectiveness of the service, and the reduction of unsafe sexual risk behaviors by youth."
- "Over a three-year period, the provincial health department, together with two local NGOs, will test and compare in terms of reduced STIs and in terms of cost-effectiveness two approaches to implementing a 100 percent condom use policy in brothels. One approach will be tested in Puerto Plata and the other in Santo Domingo. At each site, all commercial sex establishments will be enrolled in the study. All sex workers and brothel owners will receive extensive group counseling on the need to use condoms. Educational materials will be made widely available and condoms will be distributed free of charge."

- "Over a three-year period, researchers at Kenyatta National Hospital will develop and implement a comprehensive training program for staff, and an HIV/AIDS voluntary counseling and testing service for pregnant women attending the antenatal unit at the hospital. Women who test positive will be offered antiretroviral medication plus breast milk substitutes. The effect of these activities will be measured in terms of reduced rates of mother-to-child HIV transmission, cost-effectiveness, acceptability to staff, and participation by pregnant women and their partners."
- "Over a four-year period, the Amber and Victoria Gold Mining Company, together with three local NGOs, will implement a comprehensive STI control program among miners and sex workers. This program will consist of behavior change communication using peer educators, condom promotion and distribution through social marketing, and STI services, including periodic presumptive treatment among sex workers. The effect of these activities will be measured in terms of reduced prevalence of STIs among miners and sex workers, greater condom use, increased safe sex practices, and increased knowledge about HIV/AIDS transmission."

Comments on the Examples

Note that, in each of these objectives, the investigator promises to undertake **a specific activity**: to develop a program activity and measure the effect; to test and compare two different program strategies for implementing a 100 percent condom program; to develop, implement, and measure the effect of an MTCT program; and to implement and measure the effect of an STI reduction program among miners and sex workers. The situation or context involved in the research is also specified. **Who** will conduct the study, **where** it will be conducted, and **when** it will be conducted are stated. Finally, and most important, the key variables of interest are indicated, such as accep-

tance by youth of VCT, cost-effectiveness, sexual risk reduction, reduction of STIs, reduced transmission of HIV from mother to child, and increased condom use.

Each of these variables needs to be carefully defined in operational terms later in the proposal, but at least as stated here in the immediate objectives, they indicate the focus of the proposed research and some of the key variables that will be examined.

Hypotheses

A hypothesis is a statement about an expected relationship between two or more variables that permits empirical testing. While ultimate objectives identify the anticipated contributions arising from a study, and immediate objectives (stated in behavioral terms) specify what will be done or measured in the study, hypotheses specify the **expected relationship** among the variables. Hypothesis statements are most appropriate for field intervention or evaluative studies. Diagnostic or exploratory studies do not normally require hypothesis statements because they generally do not test relationships between variables.

Study hypotheses serve to direct and guide the research. They indicate the major independent and dependent variables of interest. They suggest the type of data that must be collected and the type of analysis that must be conducted in order to measure the relationship among the variables.

A single hypothesis might state that variable A is **associated** with variable B, or that variable A **causes** variable B. Sometimes a hypothesis will specify that, **under conditions X, Y, and Z,** variable A is associated with or causes variable B. A well-written hypothesis focuses the attention of the researcher on specific variables.

When writing hypothesis statements, it is important to keep in mind the distinction between **independent** and **dependent variables**. An independent variable **causes, determines,** or **influences** the dependent variable. An example of the basic relationship between these two types of variables is shown in Figure 4.1. This model shows a **direct relationship**. In other words, whenever the independent variable changes, the dependent variable changes. The dependent variable **depends** on the independent variable.

FIGURE 4.1
A direct relationship between independent and dependent variables

| Independent variables | → Cause, determine, or influence → | Dependent variables |

This type of direct relationship is usually the model used to develop study hypotheses, but in some cases, a study will hypothesize a model in which the relationship is indirect. The independent variable acts on the dependent variable through **intervening variables**. These intervening variables serve to either increase or decrease the effect the independent variable has on the dependent variable.

Intervening variables are sometimes referred to as **test** or **control** variables. In longitudinal field experiments, the design of the study (with random assignment of cases to experimental and comparison areas) usually controls the intervening variables. In cross-sectional surveys, intervening variables are measured and then controlled in the statistical analysis. Many HIV/AIDS behavioral and epidemiological research studies are based on a model that includes intervening variables (see Figure 4.2).

FIGURE 4.2
Intervening variables

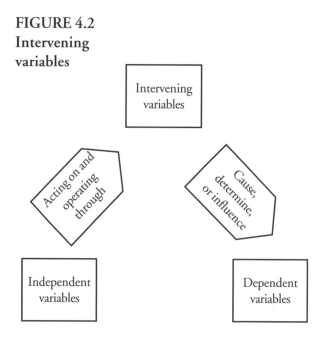

For example, in an effort to increase condom use (the dependent variable), an HIV/AIDS program might initiate a large information, education, and communication campaign (the independent variable). Alone and by itself, an IEC program cannot increase condom use. The program must act on and operate through a set of intervening variables, which in turn cause, determine, or influence condom use. There may be many of these intervening variables, but the most likely ones that might be influenced by an IEC program would be people's knowledge about HIV transmission, their attitudes about the use of condoms, their sexual risk behaviors, and their beliefs about their vulnerability to AIDS. A possible research model for an evaluation study of the effects of an IEC program is shown in Figure 4.3.

FIGURE 4.3
The effects of intervening variables in an IEC program

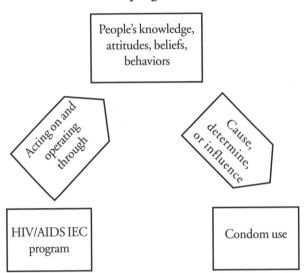

In HIV/AIDS operations research, the hypotheses of most importance usually are those that consider program activities as the independent variable. The HIV/AIDS program input, such as an IEC effort, a voluntary counseling and testing service, an STI prevention program, or a condom promotion program, is the independent variable. The objective of the research is to determine the extent to which the independent variable affects the dependent variable. The dependent variable is usually the central concern of a research proposal's problem statement. The intervening variables are important because they tend to either increase or decrease the strength of the relationship between the program (the independent variable) and the outcome effect (the dependent variable). It is therefore important to gather information on possible intervening variables.

Most research studies will examine many independent variables and many intervening variables but only a few dependent variables. In writing study hypotheses, always think in terms of the expected relationship between variables. Think first about the central problem your study will address (the dependent variable). Next, consider what factor or factors (the independent variables) might cause, determine, or influence the dependent variable. Finally, ask yourself if the relationship between the independent and dependent variables is direct or indirect through a set of intervening variables.

Examples of Hypotheses

- Students who participate in a school-based life skills education program will have more knowledge about HIV risk behaviors and prevention practices and more positive attitudes about safe sex practices than comparable students who do not participate in the life skills program. As a result, they will be more likely to delay sexual debut and use condoms than comparable students who do not participate in the life skills program.

- PLHA who receive comprehensive counseling on antiretroviral therapy that includes discussion of the side effects and their management before ARV treatment begins are more likely to adhere effectively to treatment after a year than PLHA who have not received counseling on ARVs before they begin therapy.

- Peer educators who receive a five-week, field-based training course will have higher knowledge about HIV/AIDS and be more highly motivated than peer educators who have received a three-week, classroom-based training course. As a result, work performance of the peer educators who have been trained for five weeks will be significantly higher than peer educators who have received a three-week training course that was based in the classroom.

- Higher levels of peer educator work performance will lead to higher rates of consistent condom use among youth.

- Voluntary counseling and testing programs that are linked to community-based HIV/AIDS organizations will be more successful in reducing stigma and discrimination directed at PLHA than VCT programs not linked to community-based HIV/AIDS organizations.

- Reduced levels of stigma and discrimination against PLHA will lead to more people seeking voluntary counseling and testing.

- Community-based HIV/AIDS organizations that actively involve PLHA in the planning and implementation of programs will be more likely to achieve their objectives than similar organizations that do not involve PLHA in the planning and implementation of programs.

- Dual protection programs that focus on counseling women together with their male partners will be more successful than dual protection programs that focus only on counseling women.

Comments on the Examples

Note that in each hypothesis there is a statement of an expected relationship between two or more variables. In the first hypothesis, the expected relationship is between attending a life skills education program (the independent variable) and knowledge about HIV/AIDS, and more positive attitudes toward safe sex (the intervening variables). These intervening variables are then hypothesized to have a relationship with the delay of sexual debut and on condom use (the dependent variables). In the second hypothesis, the relationship is between comprehensive counseling on ARVs (the independent variable) and adherence to ARV treatment after a year (the dependent variable).

The third and fourth hypotheses go together. In the third hypothesis, the relationship is between a five-week, field-based training program (the independent variable) and greater knowledge about HIV/AIDS and higher motivation (the intervening variables). These intervening variables are then hypothesized to have an effect on work performance (the dependent variable). Hypothesis 4 carries this causal process one step further by suggesting that work performance (which is now the independent variable) will have an effect on condom use (the dependent variable). Taken together, the model for these two hypotheses would look like Figure 4.4.

FIGURE 4.4

A model for two hypotheses about the effect of a peer educator training program on higher rates of condom use

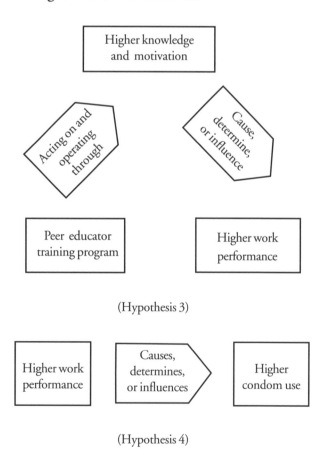

(Hypothesis 3)

(Hypothesis 4)

Similarly, hypotheses 5 and 6 go together. In hypothesis 5, VCT programs linked to community-based organizations (the independent variable) are hypothesized to reduce stigma and discrimination against PLHA (the dependent variable). In hypothesis 6, reduced stigma and discrimination become the independent variable, and use of VCT centers becomes the dependent variable.

For all the hypotheses listed in the examples, the important point is that they show a relationship between an independent and a dependent variable, and it is this relationship that is tested empirically through a research study.

To summarize, all research studies should include a statement of (1) ultimate objectives, (2) immediate objectives, and (3) hypotheses (except in the case of purely exploratory or descriptive studies). Each of these statements serves a different purpose:

1. **Ultimate objectives** state the **anticipated (hoped-for) contributions** of the study.
2. **Immediate objectives** state **what will be done** in the study.
3. **Hypotheses** state the **expected relationship** between two or more variables.

What To Do: Writing Ultimate Objectives, Immediate Objectives, and Hypotheses

1. List the major variables of your study under the headings: Independent Variables and Dependent Variables. Intervening variables can be listed under both headings. The dependent variable(s) should relate directly to your problem statement.

2. Review the list of dependent variables and then write a statement of ultimate objectives that relates to them. Ask yourself, "If I knew the factors that caused, determined, or influenced the dependent variable(s), how would this knowledge help policymakers, program administrators, or others?" How will the results from the study help improve service delivery, improve training programs, or assist in the design of educational materials? In other words, what are the anticipated contributions of the study?

3. Now write the immediate objectives for your study. Focus your attention on the specific actions that you will perform. Exactly what do you plan to do? What variables do you plan to measure? Write behavioral objectives that answer the following questions:

   - Who will do?
   - How much of what?
   - To whom?
   - When?
   - Where?
   - For what purpose?

4. Finally, write the hypotheses that your study will test. Review once again your list of independent and dependent variables. How are these variables related? Are there special conditions that must be present before they are related? Write hypothesis statements in **positive,** not negative, terms. Write a hypothesis for each major relationship that you expect to test in your study.

CHAPTER 5

INTERVENTION DESCRIPTION

If your study includes an intervention, such as a test of a new training procedure or a comparison of two new approaches to service delivery, you need to fully describe the nature of the intervention in your proposal. You should elaborate on the questions you answered when writing the immediate objectives, namely, **who will do, how much of what, to whom, when, where,** and **for what purpose.**

More specifically, it is important to answer in some detail the following questions:

Who will be responsible for implementing the intervention? Indicate the organization(s) that will be responsible for implementation and their capacity to implement the study. Also, indicate the categories of people (for example, nurses, doctors, midwives, or field motivators) who will be involved and the role of each of these persons.

Where will the intervention activities take place? Be as specific as you can about the actual location of the study intervention. Will the intervention be implemented in an entire province, in one district, in ten villages, in 30 factories, or in four clinics? Be sure to mention the location of the study sites.

What activities will be initiated? You should describe the sequence of events that will take place. For example, a study intervention might start with the training of peer educators. The nature and duration of the training should be described. Next, a series of village meetings might be held. The frequency and purpose of these meetings should be noted. Finally, the educators will visit at least five homes each day for a period of one year. The purpose of the visits and the expected activities during the visits should be described. In describing the activities that will be implemented, it is important to indicate the level or intensity of each activity.

For example, if the intervention being tested is an IEC campaign, you should describe in detail the nature of the campaign. Indicate the type of media that will be used (television, radio, newspapers, pamphlets, wall posters, group meetings, plays, or songs). Mention the intensity of the media effort (100 wall posters, 1,000 pamphlets, three radio spots per day for six months, one TV program a week for three months). Specify who will produce the posters, pamphlets, radio and TV scripts, plays, songs, and so forth; what kind of training (if any) will be needed; and what special equipment will be required.

Example of a Study Intervention Description

"An Experimental Operations Research Study in The Gambia to Provide HIV/AIDS Education and Condoms in the Workplace"

Study Intervention Sites

This employment-based HIV/AIDS prevention study will be implemented by The Gambia Rotary Club. All employment sites will be located in and around Banjul. Potential sites will include those with at least 100 employees, of whom 20 or more are female workers (the Rotary Club wants to increase women's access to HIV/AIDS education and condoms). It is estimated that some 25 employment sites will meet these criteria and approximately 15 to 20 of these will agree to participate in the project. Thus, at a minimum, the 15 employment sites should have approximately 1,500 employees (15 sites x 100 employees), of whom 300 (15 x 20) should be female employees. In fact, the number of total employees and female employees is expected to be far greater.

Although The Gambia does not have large industrial enterprises, several of them employ more than 100 workers, including breweries, hotels, the port authority, and commercial farm operations. The Rotary Club has already contacted a number of work sites to determine potential interest in participating in the study, and all enterprises contacted have expressed an interest.

To ensure active and informed participation in the study, site visits and seminars will be organized by the Rotary Club for management and workers' representatives before the study intervention begins. The purpose of the seminars will be to outline the project design and objectives and to convince management of the short- and long-term advantages of participating in the activity. The seminars will be organized in collaboration with the Ministry of Labor and the Department of Medicine and Health.

Study Activities

Employment sites willing to participate in the project will be stratified on the basis of the number of employees. Two strata will be created: (1) employment sites with 149 employees, and (2) sites with 150 or more employees. From within each stratum, employment sites will be randomly assigned to one of three groups: stationary services, mobile services, and the control group, which will receive the usual company services. The activities to be initiated in the two experimental groups are described below.

STATIONARY SERVICE SITES

At the stationary service sites, one peer educator for every 40 workers will be selected by the workers themselves, with the approval of management. The distributors will receive a total of ten days of training on sexually transmitted infections, including HIV/AIDS. Five days of training will be completed before the intervention phase of the study begins. The remaining five days of training will be spread over the duration of the intervention period, one day at a time.

The primary job of the distributor will be to provide fellow workers with information on STIs, sell condoms on a commission basis, and make referrals to the Department of Health clinics for STI treatment and voluntary counseling and testing for HIV. Each distributor will be given three bright-colored T-shirts with the Rotary Club logo to help other workers identify them. In addition, they will be given a bag to store condoms and record-keeping forms.

The stationary service sites will receive monthly supervisory visits from a Department of Health educator, who is a trained midwife. One of the primary functions of the supervisor will be to sell the distributor condoms for resale to clients and to provide support to the peer educator. The distributor will be allowed to keep half of the final sale price. Currently, a strip of four condoms sells for approximately 12 cents. Thus, for each strip of four condoms sold, the distributor earns 6 cents and the Department of Health recovers 6 cents.

In addition to resupplying the distributors, the midwife will also hold group meetings with the workers to discuss STIs, safe-sex education, and VCT. Work site managers will be requested to allow 15 minutes of work time every two weeks for educational sessions. The workers will be asked to give an equal amount of time for these educational sessions during their work break.

MOBILE SERVICE SITES

Work sites assigned to the mobile services group will receive visits every two weeks by a Department of Health educator/midwife. She will hold group meetings with the workers to discuss STIs, including HIV/AIDS, safe sex, VCT, and sources of condoms. Work site managers will be requested to allow 15 minutes of work time every two weeks for educational sessions. The workers will be asked to give an equal amount of time for these educational sessions during their work break. In addition, the educator/midwife will sell condoms. The full price of the sale will be reimbursed to the health department. As in the stationary service sites, the midwife/educator will make appointments for workers at the nearest health department clinics for STI diagnosis and treatment, VCT, and/or other desired services.

Recruitment and Training of Field Staff

The Department of Health has a cadre of educator/midwives who are responsible for carrying out HIV/AIDS information, education, and communication programs. From this cadre, four will be selected to work on this OR study. They will be responsible for conducting the field activities, scheduling the on-site education visits, monitoring condom distribution activities, and collecting routine service statistics on sales and the number of referrals to clinics. They will also provide in-service education and training for the work site distributors. Two educator/midwives will be responsible for the activities in the stationary service group, and the other two will be responsible for those in the mobile service group.

Although the educator/midwives have already been trained in the substantive areas of HIV/AIDS prevention, a short orientation program on this OR study will be organized for them. This orientation will provide an opportunity to discuss the design of the project and to review the requirements and responsibilities of the educators and workplace distributors. The midwives will be randomly assigned to a pair of study groups. Each pair will include one mobile site group and one stationary site group.

A member of the Rotary Club staff will serve as a research assistant. The research assistant will interview workers and collect service statistics and other relevant data from the workplaces. Training for the research assistant will be provided by the Department of Health.

The principal investigator will coordinate recruitment of workplace distributors with assistance from the educator/midwives. Employees in the work sites will be encouraged to participate in selecting the peer educator for their site. Selection criteria will be provided to assist them in identifying suitable peer educators. Those selected should show an interest in becoming involved in the project, demonstrate positive attitudes toward HIV and STI prevention, and be respected by workers and management.

Peer educators will participate in a required initial five-day training session and in a subsequent series of five one-day training sessions to be conducted by the Department of Health. These training sessions will be scheduled on days that are convenient for the participants and the trainers.

What To Do: Intervention Description

1. Be as detailed and complete as possible in describing the study intervention.

2. Be sure that the theoretical rationale for selecting the intervention is clear.

3. Describe the activities in the order in which they will occur.

4. Be sure your description of the intervention answers the three basic questions:

   - Who will be responsible for implementation?
   - Where will the intervention take place?
   - What activities will be initiated at what level of intensity?

CHAPTER 6

OPERATIONAL DEFINITIONS

After formulating the study objectives and hypotheses and describing fully the study intervention, the next step in the research process is to define operationally the key variables and terms of the study. Operational definitions serve two essential purposes: (1) They establish the rules and procedures the research investigator will use to measure the key variables of the study, and (2) they provide unambiguous meaning to terms that otherwise might be interpreted in different ways. Every research proposal must include operational definitions of major variables and terms.

Operational Definitions of Variables

Suppose that a dependent variable of a study is knowledge about how HIV/AIDS is transmitted. Before this variable can be measured, it is necessary first to establish the operational procedures that specify how the measurement will be made and at the same time define what the researcher means by the words "knowledge about how HIV/AIDS is transmitted." This variable must be defined in terms of events that are **observable by the senses** and therefore measurable.

The observable events serve as an **indicator** of the variable, knowledge about HIV/AIDS transmission. Alone and by itself, knowledge is not observable by the senses. It is an abstract concept. You cannot touch knowledge, see it, smell it, taste it, or hear it. What is needed is an observable event that can be measured and that **indicates** knowledge. Usually, such an indicator of knowledge in an HIV/AIDS study is based on a series of questions. For example, you might ask a respondent, "Do you know how a person can become infected with AIDS?" "Please list all the ways you know a person can get AIDS." "Can a person get AIDS from a mosquito bite?" "Can HIV/AIDS be transmitted through a mother's breast milk?" Each of these questions indicates whether the respondent knows about certain aspects of HIV/AIDS transmission. Asking a question and hearing a response is an observable event that can be measured.

A research study might ask ten HIV/AIDS knowledge questions. Each time a respondent gives an answer that indicates knowledge about HIV/AIDS transmission, the researcher could record a score of one. Every time an answer is given that does not indicate knowledge about HIV/AIDS transmission, the researcher could record a score of 0. For each respondent, the researcher could then add the total number of correct answers to the ten questions and create a HIV/AIDS knowledge score. This score would range from 0 correct answers to ten correct answers. Persons with a score of 0 would be operationally defined as having no knowledge about HIV/AIDS transmission. Persons with a score of ten would be operationally defined as having a high level of knowledge about HIV/AIDS transmission. In your research proposal, the operational definition of knowledge might appear as:

Knowledge about HIV/AIDS transmission	=	The number of correct answers a respondent gives to ten questions on HIV/AIDS transmission.

This is not the only way the variable could be defined operationally. You might wish to establish categories of HIV/AIDS knowledge, distinguishing between those respondents who have high HIV/AIDS knowledge, medium knowledge, low knowledge, and no knowledge. Each of these levels is a category of the variable, and each category requires an operational rule that tells you how to assign any given respondent to the category. One way of operationally defining the categories might be as follows:

High knowledge	=	Correct responses to eight or more of the ten questions.
Medium knowledge	=	Correct responses to between four and seven of the ten questions.
Low knowledge	=	Correct responses to between one and three of the ten questions.
No knowledge	=	No correct answers to any of the ten questions.

Note that the four categories of the variable are **mutually exclusive**, that is, they do not overlap. According to the operational rules established, a person cannot be placed in the category "High Knowledge" and at the same time be placed in the "Medium," "Low," or "No" category. The categories are also **totally inclusive**. There are only four categories. There is no fifth, sixth, or seventh category that a respondent might fit into.

In some instances, you may not want to be quite so specific in defining the categories of a variable before data collection. Sometimes it is preferable to determine the category "cutting points" of a variable after data have been collected and the response distribution for the variable has been examined. As a general rule, it is best to have approximately an equal number of respondents in each category. Thus, in the example above, each of the four categories of the variable—knowledge about HIV/AIDS transmission—should have approximately 25 percent of the respondents in the study population.

If it is necessary to examine the response distribution of a variable before the procedures for establishing categories can be determined, then in the operational definition section of a study proposal the category names can be specified, but you should include a note indicating that each category will consist of approximately equal numbers of respondents.

All variables must have at least two or more categories, or they are not variables but instead are constants. Whenever you are operationally defining a variable, it is always better to divide the variable into many categories instead of just a few. In the examples given above, the variable knowledge about HIV/AIDS transmission ranges from 0 to ten. That range gives a total of 11 categories.

Subsequently, in the second example shown below, we collapsed these 11 categories into just four categories consisting of high, medium, low, and no knowledge. If we wanted to, we could go even further and collapse the four categories into just two:

| Knowledge of HIV/AIDS transmission | = | A correct response to one or more of the ten questions. |
| No knowledge of HIV/AIDS transmission | = | No correct answers to any of the ten questions. |

If you start with many categories, it is always easy to collapse these down to just a few. But do not make the mistake of starting with just a few categories, because subsequently you cannot expand them. Collapsing the categories of a variable is usually done after data collection has been completed and the frequency distribution of the variable has been examined. Sometimes it is possible to determine the categories of a variable on the basis of a good questionnaire pretest.

Examples of Operationally Defined Variables

Condom use	=	The reported use of a condom at the last act of intercourse.
Frequent condom use	=	The reported use of a condom during the last five or more acts of intercourse.
Peer educator performance	=	Any peer educator who holds at least one group meeting on HIV/AIDS per month or visits at least two homes of PLHA per month.
Modern village	=	Any village that has three or more of the following facilities: electricity, a government health clinic, a paved road within half a mile, a primary school, a bank, a post office, irrigation for 50 percent or more of the farmland.

Operational Definitions of Terms

Recall that a hypothesis is a statement about an expected relationship between two or more variables. Just as it is necessary to define variables operationally, it is also necessary to operationally define the terms that indicate the nature of the relationship between the variables. For example, in many hypothesis statements, you will find such terms as those shown below:

more than	greater than
less than	larger than
higher than	bigger than
lower than	smaller than

You are also likely to see in hypothesis statements such words as these:

safer	significant
acceptable	expanded
improved	increased

Each of these terms can have a variety of meanings, so each requires an operational definition for the research proposal. The basic problem with such terms as *more than* or *less than* or *increased* is that they suggest a comparison but do not indicate the standard for the comparison. We need to know how much more and how much less and increased by how much.

Suppose a study has the following simple hypothesis:

A five-week, field-based training program will increase the knowledge about HIV/AIDS transmission among peer educators who have taken the program.

In this example, the training program is the independent variable. In the hypothesis, this variable is already defined, at least partially, as five weeks long and field-based. Knowledge about HIV/AIDS transmission is the dependent variable. We already have defined this variable as the number of correct responses to ten questions. What remains to be done is to define the term *increase*. If you do not define this term, you will find it impossible to know when the hypothesis has been proved or disproved. In other words, you need a standard of comparison that will tell you *increase by how much*. One way to define *increase* might be the following:

Increase = Among peer educators, a mean HIV/AIDS knowledge score on the post-training test that is significantly greater ($p < .05$) than the mean HIV/AIDS knowledge score of a control group of peer educators who did not participate in the training program.

Note that this operational definition not only tells us the meaning of increase but also gives us the procedures that will be used to measure the increase. The mean HIV/AIDS knowledge score of peer educators (in an experimental group) will be compared against the mean HIV/AIDS knowledge score of a control group. The hypothesis will be accepted only if the mean score of the peer educators in the experimental group is greater than and significantly different from the mean score of the control group. To be absolutely clear, we also should define the word *significantly*:

Significantly = A probability equal to or greater than .95 that the mean score of the peer educators in the experimental group is higher than the control group mean score.

To summarize, operational definitions establish the rules and procedures an investigator plans to use to measure and give meaning to variables and terms. The operational definition identifies indicators that are **observable events**. We must be able to ask a question, hear a response, see a behavior, record an action, and measure an attribute. The definition establishes categories for variables. The categories must be **mutually exclusive** and **totally inclusive**. Operational definitions also establish the **standard of comparison** the investigator will use to either accept or reject a hypothesis.

What To Do: Writing Operational Definitions

1. Write an operational definition for each variable on your list of independent and dependent variables.

2. Write an operational definition for each **term** (such as greater than, less than, increased, and significant) used to indicate the nature of the relationship between variables.

3. For each definition you write, ask yourself:

   - Are the rules and procedures for measuring the variables clear?
   - Have mutually exclusive and totally inclusive categories for the variables been established?
   - Is the standard of comparison clear for each term?

CHAPTER 7

INTERVENTION STUDY DESIGNS

Reliability and Validity

This chapter describes how to develop a study design to measure the impact of your intervention. A study design is the investigator's plan of action for answering the research questions. The objective in selecting a study design is to minimize possible errors and bias by maximizing the **reliability** and **validity** of the data.

Reliability refers to the consistency, stability, or dependability of the data. Whenever an investigator measures a variable, he or she wants to be sure that the measurement provides dependable and consistent results. A reliable measurement is one that if repeated a second time will give the same results as it did the first time. If the results are different, then the measurement is unreliable.

In surveys, reliability problems commonly result when the respondents do not understand the question, are asked about something they do not clearly recall, or are asked about something of little relevance to them. For example, a sex worker may not be able to recall the number of partners he or she has had, and a man who is not interested in using condoms is unlikely to give a reliable answer to a question about how much he would be willing to pay for a package of three colored condoms. Similarly, data obtained from service statistics and clinical forms and records can be unreliable if providers fail to record information or make frequent errors in categorizing services and treatments given to clients.

Validity refers to data that are not only reliable but also true and accurate. Put another way, validity is the extent to which a measurement does what it is supposed to do. If a measurement is valid, it is also reliable. But if it is reliable, it may or may not be valid. For example, suppose an investigator asks a respondent, "How old are you?" and the respondent replies, "I am 60 years old." The investigator then asks a second question to check on the consistency or dependability of the age measurement: "In what month and year were you born?" The respondent replies, "In September 1941." If it is now February 2002, the investigator calculates that, in fact, the respondent is 60 years old.

In this example, two questions have been asked. Each is designed to determine how old the respondent is, and each question gives the same results. The results are consistent, stable, and dependable, and are therefore reliable. But suppose later on the investigator happens to see the respondent's birth certificate, which shows that the true date of birth was September 1938. The investigator then concludes that, although the first two questions gave reliable results, they did not give valid or true results.

Researchers distinguish between two types of validity: **internal** and **external**. **Internal validity** refers to situations in which you find that your measurements are true and accurate and you can answer with confidence that a particular experimental intervention actually made or did not make a difference in a particular geographic setting with a particular population group at a particular time in history.

But a study with high internal validity may not have high external validity. **External validity** refers to the extent to which the results of a study can be generalized to other settings or groups. For example, if a certain intervention is successful in reducing unsafe sexual behavior in Uganda, will the same intervention have the same results in Brazil?

Will an intervention that was effective with heterosexuals also be effective with homosexuals? If the answer is "yes," the study is said to have high external validity, that is, the study results can be generalized to other settings and other populations. In the following section, we first discuss the problem of internal validity, and subsequently discuss the problem of external validity.

Threats to Validity

When selecting a research design, one criterion to use is the extent to which the design controls for threats to validity. In other words, a researcher wants a design that will give true and accurate information and avoid confounding factors that might invalidate the study. At a minimum, the researchers want a design that will allow them to know that an intervention actually made a difference in a particular setting, that is, a design with high internal validity. While there are many confounding factors, some common threats to validity are explained below.

History

Sometimes events occur during the life of a project that tend to either increase or decrease the expected outcomes. These events are called **history effects**. The events are not part of the research project, nor are they a planned or anticipated part of the study but events that are outside the study. They just happen, and they produce an effect that influences the study results.

Suppose that an evaluation is conducted to determine the effect an HIV/AIDS information campaign has on people's knowledge of and attitudes about HIV/AIDS. A pre-campaign survey might be conducted, and the results compared with post-campaign survey results. The comparison might indicate substantial increases in people's knowledge about HIV/AIDS and more tolerant attitudes toward people living with HIV/AIDS. The evaluator probably would conclude that the campaign was a success and its objectives fulfilled.

But suppose that during the campaign the president of the country made a major radio and TV address to the nation on the subject of HIV/AIDS prevention and the problems faced by PLHA. The question arises: Was it the campaign that produced the increases in knowledge and changes in attitudes, was it the president's address, or could it be both? The president's address represents a history effect. Thus, unless there is some way in the study design to control for this effect, the contribution of the campaign cannot be distinguished from the history effect of the president's speech.

Selection

A very common threat to validity occurs whenever the people selected for the control group differ greatly from the people selected for the experimental group. For example, suppose you wish to test the hypothesis that voluntary counseling and testing programs will be more successful in reaching young people if they are offered in the context of health, educational, and social services than if they are offered in the traditional context of health services alone. To find out if the combined services approach is more effective than the traditional approach in increasing the number of persons less than 25 years of age who are receiving VCT, you would inaugurate the combined services approach in one district (the experimental district) and the traditional services approach in another district (the control district). After one year, you would evaluate the approaches in terms of the proportion of young people who have received VCT.

Suppose the evaluation shows that a significantly greater proportion of young people in the combined services district than in the traditional services district have received VCT. In this situation, you might conclude that the combined program was more successful than the traditional

program. But when you check further, you find that there are large differences in the characteristics of young people in the two districts. In the experimental district, they tend to be better educated, more urban, and better off economically than young people in the control district. Because of these differences, young people in the experimental district may be more likely than youth in the control district to accept VCT, whether or not counseling and testing is offered in the context of additional educational and social services.

Once again, the question of validity arises. What is the true effect of the combined program? If young people in both districts were in fact similar, it might be possible to answer this question. But because there were initial differences, the effect of the combined program cannot be distinguished from the initial differences in the groups selected.

Testing

Earlier measurements can affect the results of later measurements. In operations research, testing can be an important confounding factor when changes in knowledge or behavior are being studied over time. Training program evaluators know that whenever a pretest is given, it tends to have an effect on the posttest results. Because trainees given a pretest are likely to remember some of the questions and some of the errors they made when they take the posttest, they are likely to do somewhat better on the posttest than they did on the pretest. Better performance on the posttest might have nothing to do with training. It might be due to the practice gained on the pretest.

Repeated testing can also affect results by altering an individual's response to the testing situation itself. For example, in a longitudinal study of risk behaviors, respondents may be more impatient the second or third time they are asked the same questions than they were the first time and thus may not answer questions as completely and accurately as they did during the first interview.

Instrumentation

Whenever a measurement instrument (such as a questionnaire) is changed between the pretest and the posttest, this change is likely to result in an effect that is independent of any effect caused by the intervention. For example, if knowledge of HIV/AIDS is measured on the pretest by the question, "Have you ever heard about HIV/AIDS?" and then on the posttest by the question, "Can you name three sexually transmitted diseases?" it is very likely that there will be a difference in the percentage of people with "knowledge." The difference may be due to the change in the questionnaire instrument.

Similarly, an instrumentation effect may be involved when interviewers become more experienced. An experienced interviewer may obtain more complete information from a respondent than an inexperienced interviewer. The additional information obtained may be due to the interviewer becoming more skilled in asking questions or observing events, not to the effect of a program intervention. Changes in the way information is collected or changes in the data collection instrument can thus result in a threat to validity.

Maturation

Over time, people change. In longitudinal studies, particularly those that extend over a period of years, it is not unusual to find that respondents become more experienced, more knowledgeable, and, of course, older. In other words, people mature over time. The maturation process can produce changes that are independent of the changes a program intervention is designed to produce. If a questionnaire is given to a group of participants in an abstinence program two years after program completion, they will very likely report more sexual partners than they did before they entered the program. An evaluator would probably be mistaken in concluding that the program had the effect of actually increasing sexual

experience. The results are most likely due just to a maturation effect, another threat to validity.

Differential Mortality

In cohort studies (also called panel longitudinal studies) where the same group of people are followed over time, there is almost always some dropout or loss of cases. It is often impossible to locate for a second survey all the same people who were interviewed in the first survey. Some cases will be lost to follow-up. If the people who cannot be contacted are very different from those who can be contacted, great differences are likely between the results of the first and second surveys. These differences may be due to the loss of cases rather than to the effect of a program intervention.

Regression to the Mean

There is a tendency for a person or group who scored at the extreme high end of a range of scores to achieve a lower score on a subsequent test or measurement and, conversely, for those scoring at the extreme low end to achieve a higher score on subsequent measurements. This phenomenon is known as regression to the mean.

In operations research, regression to the mean is a concern when the study focuses on changing program components at the low or high end of the performance range. For example, we may decide that peer educators who scored in the lowest 10 percent on an HIV/AIDS knowledge test should be retrained to improve their work. After retraining, the scores of the poor performers improve. But was the improvement due to the training or to regression to the mean? In our group of low-scoring educators, one person may have been sick on the day she took the test. Another may have had her test graded wrong. A third may have forgotten to turn over the test paper and thus failed to answer half of the questions. The second time they take the test, they are healthy, have their papers graded correctly, and answer all the questions. Hence their scores improve.

Each of the threats to validity (history, selection, testing, instrumentation, maturation, differential mortality, and regression to the mean) must be considered carefully when designing a research study. Unless controlled (accounted for), each validity threat represents a possible alternative reason that a program produced or did not produce an effect. In other words, it is always necessary to distinguish an effect that is due to a program intervention from an effect due to one of the confounding factors discussed in this section.

Types of Intervention Study Designs

In the following pages, several different types of intervention research designs are presented and discussed. They range from true experimental to non-experimental to quasi-experimental designs. The designs presented here are certainly not the only ones that exist, but they are some of the more frequently used designs in HIV/AIDS operations research. In describing each of these, we will use a common notation developed by Campbell and Stanley (1963). This notation is explained in Figure 7.1.

FIGURE 7.1
Notation for study designs

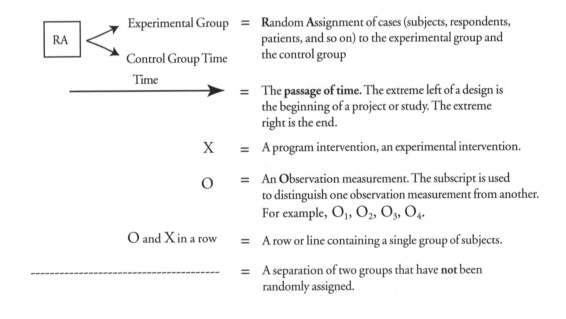

RA → Experimental Group / Control Group Time	= **R**andom **A**ssignment of cases (subjects, respondents, patients, and so on) to the experimental group and the control group
Time →	= The **passage of time.** The extreme left of a design is the beginning of a project or study. The extreme right is the end.
X	= A program intervention, an experimental intervention.
O	= An **O**bservation measurement. The subscript is used to distinguish one observation measurement from another. For example, O_1, O_2, O_3, O_4.
O and X in a row	= A row or line containing a single group of subjects.
-------------------------------------	= A separation of two groups that have **not** been randomly assigned.

Example of a Study Design

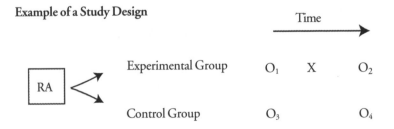

Time →

Experimental Group	O_1	X	O_2
Control Group	O_3		O_4

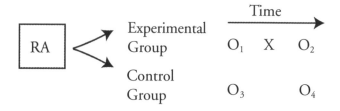

True Experimental Designs

True experimental designs are the gold standard for demonstrating causality, that is, that a change in the independent variable has produced a change in the dependent variable. The question of causality is also of vital interest to program managers, who must make decisions about continuing or scaling up interventions. Is the program activity or strategy actually helping to reduce the number of new HIV infections or are you wasting money? Does the training course produce greater knowledge among peer educators or not? The following are true experimental designs:

The example above depicts a true experimental design called the **pretest-posttest control group design**. True experiments are distinguished from other designs because all subjects are randomly assigned (RA) from a single population to the experimental and control groups. Randomized control trials (RCT) often use this true experimental design.

Random assignment of individuals (such as service providers or clients) or other study units (for example, clinics, villages, or districts) in experiments is different from **random sampling** in surveys. Random sampling ensures that the individuals in the study are truly representative of the population from which they are drawn. The purpose of **random assignment**, in contrast, is to ensure that the experimental and control groups are truly comparable to each other. Because the members of the experimental and control groups are equivalent, random assignment controls for most threats to validity.

Different techniques can be used to randomly assign study units, ranging from tossing a coin or rolling dice to using a table of random numbers or a computer-generated algorithm.

In the **pretest-posttest control group** design, both the experimental and control groups receive an initial measurement observation (the pretests O_1

and O_3). The experimental group then receives the program intervention X, but the control group does not receive this intervention. Subsequently, after the intervention period is completed, a second set of measurement observations is made (O_2 and O_4). You would expect that, since the experimental group received a special program intervention, X, O_2 would be greater than O_4. Also, since both the experimental and control cases were randomly assigned, you would expect that O_1 would be equivalent to O_3 on all factors, including such key variables as age, sex, and education. Because both groups were equivalent at the beginning of the experiment, you can feel confident in attributing any differences between the experimental and control groups that you observe at the posttest to the effect of the intervention.

Although random assignment is the preferred technique, it is not always possible for ethical, programmatic, or other reasons. For example, investigators may be interested in the effect of such variables as gender, age, or marital status on adherence to HIV therapy or on the performance of peer educators. However, none of these variables can be randomly assigned to individuals. Similarly, a Ministry of Health will probably not assign HIV prevention activities to a random group of districts, and women cannot be randomly assigned to use female condoms.

However, there are many situations in which random assignment can be used. These include experimenting with the best way to train providers and testing educational and counseling strategies, supervision, referral and logistics systems, and quality improvements. For example, a Ministry of Education might want to learn whether a brief course on HIV/AIDS prevention reduces risky sexual behavior among secondary school students. A group of 40 secondary schools could be selected for the study, with 20 randomly assigned to the experimental group (which receives the brief course) and 20 randomly assigned to the control

group (which does not receive the course). Matching cases before random assignment can make the pretest-posttest control group design even more powerful. When the unit of study is service delivery facilities or towns and villages, the operations researcher usually must rely on a small number of cases. When samples are small, it is likely that the cases will not be equivalent, even though they have been randomly assigned. In this situation, a common technique for ensuring equivalence is to match cases on a variable that is a potential threat to validity, and then randomly assign pair members to experimental and control groups. By reducing the nontreatment differences between the experimental and control groups, matching also makes it easier to achieve significance on statistical tests, as well as making it possible to reduce sample size (see chapter 8).

There are many true experimental designs other than the pretest-posttest design described above, but most are not used frequently in operations research. Consequently, we will limit the rest of our discussion to two of the more frequently used designs.

POSTTEST-ONLY CONTROL GROUP DESIGN

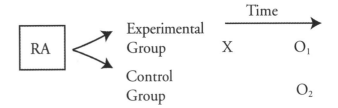

The first is the **posttest-only control group** design. This design differs from the pretest-posttest design discussed above only because it has no pretest. Since cases have been assigned randomly to the experimental and the control group, these groups are assumed to be similar before the program intervention. This design allows the investigator to measure the effect of a program intervention on the experimental group by comparing that group to the control group.

In some situations, this design could be preferable to the pretest-posttest control group design, for example, when the investigator is faced with serious time or budget constraints, when pretest data are not available, when there are concerns about a testing effect, or when a very large sample can be assigned to treatment and control groups. However, there are some drawbacks to this design. First, the posttest-only control group design does not allow an investigator to determine the extent of change within the experimental group because a baseline pretest measurement was not taken. Second, lack of a pretest measurement prevents the investigator from matching cases before random assignment to experimental and control groups.

The effectiveness of the HIV/AIDS prevention course in reducing risky sexual behavior mentioned above could be studied using either a pretest-posttest control group or a posttest-only control group design. If the former design were selected, upper-class students in all 40 schools could be asked to fill out a self-administered questionnaire about their sexual behavior during the previous six months. Schools could be matched on the basis of the pretest results and then randomly assigned to experimental and control groups. The experimental schools would teach the prevention course, and the controls would not.

Six months after the course, students would again fill out questionnaires about their sexual behavior during the past six months. The researchers would then compare the amount of change in risk behavior in both groups. If the course were effective, a greater reduction in risk behavior would be observed in the experimental than in the control group. Confidence in attributing the observed reduction to the intervention would be enhanced by the fact that the equivalence of the two groups could be demonstrated by the pretest results and matching procedure.

If the posttest-only control group design were used, students would not be asked to fill out questionnaires before randomization, and would do so only six months after the course. The researchers would then compare the amount of risk behavior in both groups. If the course were effective, less risk behavior would be found among the experimental group than in the control group. However, the researchers would be unable to demonstrate the degree of equivalence between groups at the beginning of the experiment. They would also be unable to tell Ministry of Education officials and parents how much risk reduction had occurred.

MULTIPLE TREATMENT DESIGNS

Although practical difficulties in conducting research increase with the complexity of the design, experiments examining the effects of multiple treatments are frequently used in OR studies. An advantage of multiple treatment designs is that they increase the alternatives available to managers. Two examples of multiple treatment designs are shown below.

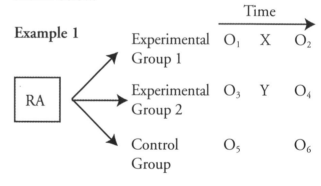

The design in Example 1 allows you to determine the relative effectiveness of different interventions (X and Y). The presence of the nontreatment control group also permits you to determine the absolute effectiveness of each intervention compared to the effectiveness of not intervening at all. Without the control group, you would not know if either X or Y were better than doing nothing at all.

Example 2

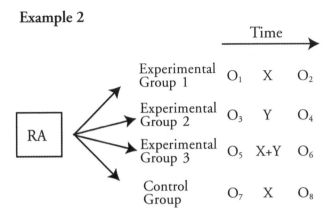

In Example 2, the multiple treatment design allows you to compare the relative effects of two interventions (X and Y) alone and in combination. The use of the control group allows you to determine whether any of the interventions are better than doing nothing. Designs like Example 2 are the preferred designs for studying the effect of integrating services. They allow you to determine the effectiveness of individual services when offered separately (X and Y) and when offered together (X + Y).

VALIDITY THREATS THAT RANDOM ASSIGNMENT DOES AND DOES NOT CONTROL

Randomization controls for selection, because every unit has an equal chance of being assigned to the experimental or control group, and it controls for the effects of testing, maturation, and history because these threats to validity should occur equally in both groups. Similarly, randomization can control for the effect of instrument bias when changes in measurement can be shown to have affected all groups equally.

Randomization does not control for differential mortality, instrument bias associated with the use of interviewers, or very small numbers of study units.

The practice of **double-blinding** in medical experiments in which neither the subject nor the investigator knows who has received the drug and who has received the placebo is an example of controlling for threats to validity associated with the conduct of the experiment itself. In OR, the experimental and control groups often are composed of only a single unit—for example, a hospital or district, or only two or three units. The small number of units sometimes makes it impossible to separate the effect of the intervention from the effect of the hospital or district where the experiment was performed.

Contamination, one of the most important problems encountered in operations research, is also not controlled by randomization. Contamination is a concern when units in close proximity are assigned to different groups. For example, if half the supervisors of a group of peer counselors in the experimental group are assigned to use a new job aid, they may share the tool with program supervisors in the control group, thereby eliminating the difference between the experimental and control groups. Avoiding possible contamination is a common reason for choosing a **quasi-experimental** rather than a **true experimental design**.

Non-experimental Designs

There are several non-experimental designs commonly used by HIV/AIDS researchers. These designs are most appropriate for collecting descriptive information or for doing small case studies. They are not recommended for evaluation studies that attempt to determine the effect or impact of a program intervention, but may be useful in diagnostic studies to determine the reasons why a problem exists.

POSTTEST-ONLY DESIGN

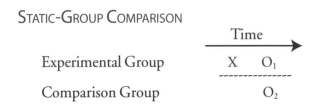

In this design, a program intervention (X) has been introduced, and sometime after its introduction, a measurement observation (O_1) is made. Since there is no control group, there is no possibility of comparing the O_1 measurement to any other measurement. All that the O_1 measurement can do is provide descriptive information. The threats to validity of history, maturation, selection, and mortality are not controlled and therefore are factors to consider before choosing this design.

This design would be appropriate if an investigator wanted to estimate, for example, the potential demand for safe-sex lectures and the characteristics of persons attending them. The treatment would be the safe-sex lecture, and the O_1 measure would consist of information collected from members of the audience at the talk. While numerous problems are associated with the posttest-only design, particularly if a comparative analysis is desired, much useful program information can be obtained if multivariate data analysis techniques are used.

PRETEST-POSTTEST DESIGN

In this design, there is still no control group, but at least there is an earlier measurement observation (O_1) that allows the investigator to examine changes over time. It is important to be aware that the pretest-posttest design is subject to several threats to validity, including history, testing, maturation, and instrumentation.

STATIC-GROUP COMPARISON

Unlike the other two designs, this one adds a comparison group. The experimental group receives a program intervention (X), followed by a measurement observation (O_1). This measurement observation is then compared against a second observation (O_2) from a control group that did not receive the program intervention. It is similar to the posttest-only comparison group design discussed above.

Note, however, that the two groups are separated by a broken line (------), which indicates that a random process was not used to create the two groups. This design might be used if patients at one clinic were used to make comparisons to patients at another clinic where a special program intervention had taken place. The primary problem with this design is the confounding factors of selection and mortality. Initially, the two groups might differ greatly on the basis of such variables as age, marital status, and education, but the extent of the difference would not be known.

Quasi-experimental Designs

As we have pointed out, in many field research situations it is simply impossible or very costly and difficult to meet the random assignment criteria of a true experimental design. At the same time, researchers want to avoid the problems of threats to validity associated with non-experimental designs. A reasonable compromise often can be made by selecting a quasi-experimental design. These designs do not have the restrictions of random assignment. At the same time, they can control for many threats to validity.

NON-EQUIVALENT CONTROL GROUP

Time →

Experimental Group	O_1	X	O_2
Control Group	O_3		O_4

The most frequently used quasi-experimental design in operations research is probably the **non-equivalent control group** design. This design is characterized by the use of a small number of collective units, such as health care facilities, administrative districts, or classrooms, each of which contains various types of individuals. The individuals in the collective units are not randomly assigned to experimental and control groups, nor are the units themselves randomly assigned (note the line between the treatment and comparison groups, which indicates that the groups were not randomly assigned).

Suppose two districts are available to test whether quality of care for illnesses related to opportunistic infection in PLHA can be improved with training in and use of standard case management guidelines for providers. Two health care facilities are available for inclusion in the OR study. One design possibility would be to randomly assign some caregivers in each facility to experimental and control groups. However, the investigators are concerned that having both experimentals and controls in the same

facility would result in contamination. That is, the controls would learn about the new guidelines from providers in the experimental group, and might begin applying them to their own patients. Under the circumstances, the best solution would be to use providers in one facility as the experimental group and providers in the other as the comparison group, thereby avoiding the risk of contamination.

The providers in one hospital could be given a pretest (O_1), followed by a brief training course in the use of the new guidelines (X) and then the posttest (O_2). For purposes of comparison, a similar group of providers from another hospital could be administered the same pretest at the same time (O_3) and could be given the same posttest (O_4). In this situation, you could use the two pretests (O_1 and O_3) to assess the extent to which the two groups of providers were truly similar. Then you would compare the two posttests (O_2 and O_4). You would expect that O_2 would be greater than O_4 because of the effect of the new guidelines.

The non-equivalent control group design is a particularly good one to use when a program intervention is introduced into one area (say, one district) and you want to compare the program effects in that district against a similar, but not necessarily equivalent, neighboring district. The non-equivalent control group design protects against history, maturation, testing, and instrumentation as sources of invalidity.

However, because the units are not randomly assigned to experimental and control groups, selection bias can never be ruled out completely. The best you can do is to compare the pretest measures to determine if the behavior of the two groups was similar before the intervention. Therefore, the researcher must pay special attention to the analysis and comparison of O_1 against O_3 (the pretest baselines). In particular, you should look for selection effects or major differences between the intervention and comparison groups that might help explain differences (or lack of differences) in the posttest O_2 and O_4 comparisons.

TIME SERIES DESIGN

Time

Experimental Group

O_1 O_2 O_3 X O_4 O_5 O_6

Time series designs are used in many different OR studies. Often they are the only feasible alternative, as in studies of mass media promotion in which the population enjoys universal access to the medium employed, making a control or comparison group impossible to find, or in situations in which only one health care facility or administrative unit is available for study.

The time series design is similar to the non-experimental pretest-posttest design except that it has the advantage of repeated measurement observations before and after the program intervention X. Suppose, for example, you find that there is no difference between O_1, O_2, and O_3, but then a sudden increase occurs between O_3 and O_4, which is subsequently maintained in O_5 and O_6. You can conclude with some degree of confidence that the sudden increase was probably due to the effect of the intervention. This type of increase might be shown in graph form, as in Figure 7.2.

FIGURE 7.2
A sudden increase in a measured variable after a program intervention

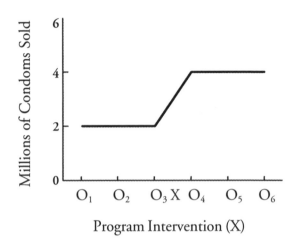

Program Intervention (X)

Suppose in this example the program intervention X is a mass media advertising campaign designed to increase condom use. Before the campaign, commercial retail audits in pharmacies (O_1, O_2, and O_3) reveal that mean monthly condom sales are about 2 million units. During the advertising campaign, mean monthly condom sales increase to 4 million units.

After the intervention, sales remain steady at the higher level at observations O_5 and O_6. The most likely explanation for the change is the campaign. But another explanation might be a history effect, such as a decrease in prices, or an instrumentation effect, such as a change in the methodology used to calculate sales by the company conducting the retail audit that happened between O_3 and O_4.

Although the possible confounding effects of history or instrumentation cannot be eliminated as an explanation for the increase in condom sales, the time series design helps the researcher avoid making mistaken or false conclusions. Suppose the researcher did not observe a sharp increase in condom sales as portrayed in Figure 7.2, but rather a steady and constant increase in sales over time as shown in Figure 7.3.

FIGURE 7.3
A constant increase in a measured variable over time regardless of a program intervention

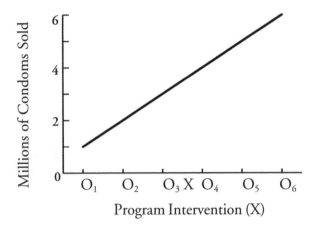

FIGURE 7.4
Regular increases and decreases in a measured variable before and after a program intervention

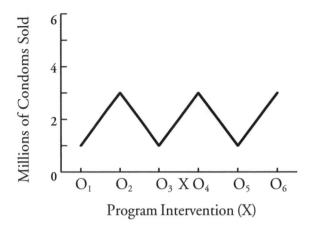

The increase is no greater between O_3 and O_4, when the intervention X took place, than it is at any other time. Obviously, in this situation the investigator could not claim that the advertising campaign made a difference. This is the advantage of the time series design. The multiple observations allow you to plot a trend. If the investigator had used the pretest-posttest design and compared only O_3 against O_4, he or she might have mistakenly concluded that the campaign had made a difference. Now examine Figure 7.4.

The trend in this example is regular and marked by alternating increases and decreases in condom sales. The advertising campaign did not seem to make a difference in this trend. But, once again, if the investigator had used a pretest-posttest design and compared only O_3 against O_4, he or she might mistakenly have concluded that the program had an impact.

The time series design is a good one to use when you have access to regularly collected information, such as monthly service statistics. You can plot the information on a graph and then note the point at which a special program intervention occurred. If there is a sudden change in the plotted line that is unusual and not similar to the trend before or after a program intervention, you can be fairly sure that the sudden change was due to the program.

Consider Figure 7.5. In this example, suppose that each month a group of pharmacies sell 3 million condoms. Measurements at O_1, O_2, and O_3 all confirm the 3 million figure. Then an advertising campaign is conducted. Suddenly, condom sales soar to 6 million per month, as shown by a retail audit conducted at time O_4. But soon after the campaign, sales drop back to the original level. The campaign clearly had an impact, but the impact did not last long. Once again, had the investigator used a pretest-posttest design and compared only O_3 against O_4, he or she would mistakenly have concluded that the campaign had an enormous impact. But the investigator would have missed the important point that the impact was only temporary.

FIGURE 7.5
Temporary impact of a program intervention

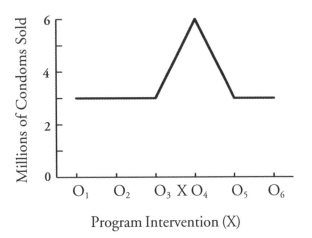

To summarize, although the time series design does not include a control group and does not control for history and instrumentation threats to validity, it does allow for a more detailed analysis of data and program impact than the pretest-posttest design because it gives information on trends before and after a program intervention. It is a particularly appropriate design to use when a researcher can make multiple measurement observations before and after a program intervention.

SEPARATE SAMPLE PRETEST-POSTTEST DESIGN

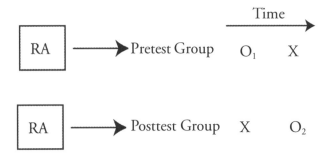

This design is an alternative to the non-experimental pretest-posttest design. The separate sample design is stronger than the pretest-posttest design because it eliminates testing as a source of invalidity. However, like the pretest-posttest design it does not control for history, maturation, mortality, or, possibly, instrumentation effects. The design involves doing a baseline pretest (O_1) with a randomly selected sample from a study population. Subsequently, a program intervention (X) is introduced, and then a posttest measurement (O_2) is made using a second randomly selected sample from the same study population. This design might be used, for example, to evaluate the effect of an information campaign on community attitudes toward PLHA or to evaluate the effect of training on peer educator knowledge.

Selecting a Study Design

Selecting an appropriate operations research study design can be tricky. It usually requires careful consideration of ethical issues and balancing technical issues against practical, financial, and administrative concerns.

Ethical Issues

The first issues to consider in selecting a research design are the ethical ones. If a particular research design results in unethical procedures, a violation of people's rights and dignity, or a denial of services that otherwise would be available, then the design should be modified or abandoned, regardless of the effect this may have on reliability, validity, time, funds, and available personnel. Indeed, if it is not possible to do an ethical study, then the study should not be done. This point cannot be compromised.

Most OR study proposals, particularly those that deal with sensitive HIV/AIDS issues, need to be sent to your organization's Institutional Review Board (IRB). The IRB will review the proposal to make sure that ethical issues are handled correctly and that the study procedures meet all the legal requirements necessary to conduct research. If your organization does not have an IRB, it is important that you send your proposal to respected individuals who are capable of reviewing it for ethical and legal issues.

Practical, Financial, and Administrative Issues

Every researcher dreams of having available for a study lots of funds, time, personnel, and a large pool of perfect study units that can be randomly assigned. Unfortunately, dreams are not reality. Most often funds are limited, time is short, personnel are few in number, and the number of units available for study is considerably less than ideal.

Obviously, these real-world conditions affect research and, in particular, the design of operations research. Available funds, time, and personnel may not permit three experimental groups and one control group. They may not allow a large and detailed baseline survey and another follow-up survey 24 months later. They also may not permit running the study intervention for 36 months. All of these practical and administrative issues unavoidably affect the selection of a research design.

Technical Issues

While the technical objective in selecting a research design is to minimize possible errors, the dynamic field setting of most operations research studies usually presents numerous threats to the reliability and validity of the study. Almost always, experimental field studies face unanticipated events, such as the closing of a service delivery center, the transfer of key personnel, a civil disturbance, a flood, or other happenings that affect the research design or change the study intervention. The effects these events have on the reliability and validity of a study are often unclear or even unknown, but they certainly can be substantial. Some of the important technical issues you should keep in mind when selecting a research design are listed below:

- Whenever possible, try to create experimental and control groups by assigning cases randomly from a single population study group. Match cases before randomly assigning them whenever you can.
- When random assignment is not possible, try to find a comparison group that is as nearly equivalent to the experimental group as possible.
- When neither a randomly assigned control group nor a similar comparison group is available, try to use a time series design that can provide information on trends before and after a program intervention.
- If a time series design cannot be used, at least try to obtain baseline (pretest) information that can be compared against post-program information (a pretest-posttest design) before a program starts.
- If baseline (pretest) information is unavailable, be aware that you will be limited in the type of analysis you can conduct. You should consider using multivariate analytic techniques.
- Always keep in mind the issue of validity. Are the measurements true? Do they do what they are supposed to do? Are there possible threats to validity (history, selecting, testing, maturation, mortality, or instrumentation) that might explain the results?

GUIDELINES FOR A "GOOD" RESEARCH DESIGN

- A good research design is an ethical research design. It is a design that does not violate people's rights and dignity and that does not deny people the quality of services they otherwise would have had available to them.
- A good research design is capable of obtaining the most reliable and valid data possible, given the constraints of funds, time, personnel, and equipment.
- A good research design is capable of measuring whatever it is that happens in a field setting, whether it is the impact of planned intervention activities or the impact of unplanned and possibly invalidating events.
- A good research design helps an investigator avoid making erroneous conclusions, such as accepting a hypothesis when in fact the hypothesis is false or rejecting a hypothesis when in fact the hypothesis is true.

External Validity in Intervention Research and the Principle of the Three Multiples

Earlier in this chapter we mentioned the issue of external validity, or "generalizability." In the experimental research tradition, external validity is demonstrated through replication. The experiment is repeated in other areas, with other populations, and by other researchers. If the results are similar to the original experiment, the intervention can be said to be generalizable to those situations in which the replications were conducted.

In program situations, however, funds and time for replication are often unavailable. Nonetheless, as much as possible, researchers should seek independent verification of their studies. It is always a good idea to keep in mind the **principle of the three multiples** whenever you are selecting a research design.

1. **Seek multiple data sources to obtain information on the same variables.**

2. **Seek multiple measurements over time on the same variables.**

3. **Seek multiple replications of the study intervention in different field settings.**

Multiple data sources serve several purposes. First, each source can provide a reliability check on the other sources. Second, each source may provide additional insights about a particular event or a relationship between events. Third, the use of multiple data sources provides the opportunity to obtain qualitative information on process that can be particularly useful in determining how and why an intervention effect was obtained or not obtained.

Multiple measurements over time of the same variables can provide information on trends before, during, and after the introduction of an intervention. This type of information can be extremely valuable for field studies. Sudden and radical deviations from past trends can be the first indication that factors extraneous to a study intervention are affecting an experimental area or population.

Multiple replications of a study intervention in different settings and by different researchers can provide information about the extent to which the intervention's effects are unique to a particular area and population or can be generalized to other areas and populations. Ideally, the use of multiple replications means that one or more follow-up studies are conducted with the same objectives and research design, but are implemented in different areas. In practice, because of time and resource constraints, this is difficult to accomplish. An alternative is to introduce the intervention in several field settings at the same time. This procedure not only provides an indication about the degree to which the intervention's impact can be generalized, but also gives some guarantee that if one experimental area is affected by floods, riots, administrative delays, strikes, or other events, at least the study can continue in the other areas.

What To Do: Designing a Study

1. The objectives of a research study determine to a large extent the type of research design required. Review the objectives of your study and consider the following questions:

   - Are you planning to evaluate a program? If your answer is yes, consider using an experimental or a quasi-experimental design.
   - Are you interested only in describing a particular event? If the event has already taken place, you can use a posttest-only design ($X O_1$) and consider multivariate analysis to examine the data. If the event has not yet taken place, you might be able to use a pretest-posttest design ($O_1 X O_2$), a time series design ($O_1 O_2 O_3 X O_4 O_5 O_6$), or a non-equivalent control group.

   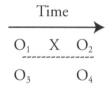

   - Will you be conducting an experiment to determine the effect of a particular approach on HIV/AIDS service delivery? If your answer is yes, you should try to obtain a randomly assigned control group or at least a comparison group that is similar to the experimental group.

2. On the basis of your answers to the questions above, diagram with O's and X's the type of design you think is most appropriate for your research study. Remember that many variations are possible for the designs presented earlier.

3. Consider the ethical implications, if any, of the design.

4. Be sure that available time and resources are adequate to implement the design. Review the list of threats to validity and determine which ones are controlled and which ones are not.

CHAPTER 8

SAMPLING

Many operations research projects depend on data that have been obtained from samples. The purpose of this chapter is to explain why researchers sample and to describe some basic sampling considerations and strategies. The chapter seeks to enable you to identify situations in which different types of sampling might be appropriate. Although it will prepare you to work with a sampling specialist, it will not make you a sampling specialist.

A sample can be thought of as a model of a larger population. A sample consists of a relatively small number of individuals or other units that are selected from a larger population according to a set of rules. For example, you may **randomly** select 100 PLHA who are part of a total population of 600 PLHA served by the outpatient clinic of Central Hospital. If you have a good model, you may be able to generalize from your sample of PLHA to all PLHA in the outpatient clinic.

Similarly, if you use a sample consisting of all types of women in the country, you may be able to generalize your results to the total population of women. The advantage of studying a sample of cases as opposed to all cases is that the research can be done more quickly, less expensively, and often more accurately than a large **census** (survey of the entire population). In fact, given limited research budgets and typically large population sizes, there is usually no alternative to sampling.

For example, you might want to evaluate the impact of a national radio campaign on the attitudes of adults toward people living with HIV/AIDS. Such a study would probably involve comparing the results of two sample surveys. The first might be a nationally representative survey of adults conducted before the campaign, and the second a survey of the same group conducted after the campaign. Similarly, if you were studying the effect of an intervention to increase dual protection among married couples, you might introduce the intervention in one district and use a matched district as a control. You would then conduct a survey that was representative of all married couples in the districts and compare the prevalence of dual protection.

There are two general types of samples: **probability (or random)** and **nonprobability samples**. The nature of your operations research study will determine which type of sampling you should use. Large-scale descriptive studies almost always use probability sampling techniques. Intervention studies sometimes use probability sampling but also frequently use nonprobability sampling. Qualitative studies almost always use nonprobability samples.

Probability Sampling

In chapter 7, we discussed experimental and quasi-experimental design techniques for controlling the internal validity of a study. Probability sampling is a technique you can use to maximize external validity or generalizability of the results of the study. Descriptive studies and large operations research intervention studies are frequently designed so that their results are as generalizable as possible.

Three factors determine how accurate a sample is as a description of a population:

1. The methods used to select the sample must not bias the sample, that is, the sample must be truly representative of the larger universe. For example, if you wanted a sample of women ages 15–49 and selected only unmarried women who are friends of the interviewers, this would be a biased sample.

2. The characteristics of the sample must be consistent with the characteristics of the population of interest (for example, if the population is unmarried women, the sample must consist of unmarried women).

3. The numerical estimates provided by the sample must accurately represent the true values in the population. For example, if the true number of condom users in a population is 30 percent and your sample estimates that it is between 35 and 45 percent, the sample is not an accurate representation of the population. However, if you estimate that the true number of condom users is between 28 and 32 percent, your sample is a fairly accurate representation of the population.

The essence of probability sampling is that each element of the larger population (that is, each couple, each field worker, or each clinic) has a **known, non-zero probability of being selected**. This is achieved through random selection of units for the sample from a list or sampling frame (see definition below). The **random process** guards against the introduction of bias into the sample by the researcher and against other types of systematic bias. The accuracy of the sampling frame is important for meeting the criterion that the characteristics of the sample be consistent with the characteristics of the total population.

A **sampling frame** is a list of the population from which the sampling units are drawn. In the rural health center example, your sampling frame would be the list of health centers maintained by the Ministry of Health that are located in rural areas. The completeness of a sampling frame is critical to the "representativeness" of a sample chosen from the frame. If the Ministry's list of clinics were out of date and did not include clinics opened after 1999, the sample would be representative only of clinics opened in 1999 or earlier, not of new clinics. Similarly, the sample frame would also be inaccurate if some health centers that had been closed in 2000 were still included on the list, or if some centers were inadvertently listed more than once.

Finally, the **sample size** must be large enough to deliver the level of accuracy or **precision** required in your estimate of the value in the total population. We will discuss five commonly used probability sampling techniques that prevent bias.

Simple Random Sampling

In simple random sampling, each element of the larger population is assigned a unique number, and a table of random numbers or a lottery technique is used to select elements, one at a time, until the desired sample size is reached. Bias is avoided because the person drawing the sample does not manipulate the lottery or random numbers table to select certain individuals.

Simple random sampling is usually reserved for use with relatively small populations with an easy-to-use sampling frame. For example, if the medical records files (the sampling frame) of 600 outpatients (the universe) are ordered consecutively from 1 to 600, it will be quite easy to draw a simple random sample of 100 outpatients. However, this procedure can be very tedious when drawing large samples.

Systematic Sampling

This is a modification of simple random sampling, which is ordinarily less time-consuming and easier to implement. The estimated number of elements in the larger population is divided by the desired sample size, yielding a **sampling interval** (let us call it n). The sample is then drawn by listing the population elements in an arbitrary order and selecting every n^{th} case, starting with a randomly selected number between 1 and n.

In the text box above, we discussed the problem of sampling rural health centers. In this example, your sampling frame would be a list of rural health centers arranged alphabetically by health center name. If your desired sample size is 285 rural health centers drawn from a universe of 2,000 rural health centers, the sampling interval is 2,000/285 = 7. You would then choose a randomly selected number between 1 and 7 as your start. If your random number is 3, the first unit selected would be the 3rd rural clinic listed in the sampling frame, the second would be the 10th (7 + 3) clinic listed, the third the 17th, and so on until the sampling frame is exhausted. Systematic sampling is useful when the units in your sampling frame are not numbered, when the elements are not numbered serially, or when the sampling frame consists of very long lists.

Stratified Sampling

Populations often consist of **strata**, or groups, that are different from each other and that consist of very different sizes. For example, rural health centers, urban health centers, and hospitals are very different kinds of establishments in most developing countries. Similarly, the proportion of urban and rural residents in a country or of HIV-positive and HIV-negative patients attending prenatal clinics are liable to be very different. To ensure that all relevant strata of the population are represented in your sample, you would use a technique called **stratified sampling**.

Stratification may be used in conjunction with either simple random sampling or systematic sampling. When stratifying, each stratum is treated as a separate population. You would arrange your sample frame by strata, and then draw a random or systematic sample from each. Estimates for each stratum are then combined to produce an estimate for the total population.

You can draw either a **proportionate** or **disproportionate** stratified sample. If it were important that the age distribution of your sample is the same as the age distribution of your population, you would draw a proportionate sample by using the same or **unified sampling** fraction for each group (for example, if your strata were ten-year age groups between ages 15 and 44, you might sample every 100th person aged 15–24, every 100th person aged 25–34, and every 100th person aged 35–44).

Proportionate stratified samples are perhaps the most commonly used type of stratified sampling. However, in HIV/AIDS operations research, you sometimes encounter situations in which strata are so different in size that it is impossible to get a needed minimum sample size. If you use a single sampling fraction, you must draw a disproportionate stratified sample. For example, if your strata are 4,000 rural health centers, 3,000 urban health centers, and 50 hospitals and you want to estimate the proportion of AIDS-related visits in each strata, you would have to use a smaller sampling fraction for hospitals than for health centers.

Cluster Sampling

Cluster sampling is the most commonly used probability sampling technique in the behavioral sciences. Cluster sampling refers to techniques in which samples are selected in two or more stages. Cluster sampling is used when it is not possible to get an adequate sampling frame for the individuals you wish to study, or when a simple random sample technique would result in a list of individuals so dispersed that it would be too costly to visit each one. The disadvantage of a cluster sample is that it increases sampling error and requires a larger sample size for reliable estimates of population characteristics. If the cost of the larger sample size outweighs the costs associated with unclustered sampling, clustering should not be used.

A **cluster** is a group of sampling units rather than an individual unit. Examples of clusters include all the AIDS patients in a hospital, all the peer educators in a district, all the women in a town, or all the children in a household. You would probably use cluster sampling to study AIDS widows. No list of AIDS widows exists, but you do have a list of households. Your strategy would be to first select a random sample of households. If the clusters contained a small number of individuals—for example, only one or two women of marriageable age per household—then you might interview all of the individual sampling elements included in the cluster. However, if the number of sampling elements per cluster is large (for example, the number of AIDS patients in a hospital), you would select a random sample of elements from within the cluster. This is referred to as **two-stage cluster sampling**.

Multi-stage Cluster Sampling

Sometimes, when populations are extremely complex, it is necessary to go beyond two stages in cluster sampling, a technique referred to as **multi-stage cluster sampling**. For example, if you do not have a list of households for your survey of AIDS widows, you might have to begin with a random sample of villages (called the **primary sampling unit** or **PSU**), and when you arrive at each village, make a list of households (called the **secondary sampling unit**) and draw a random selection of households to visit. When you arrive at a household, you would randomly select a woman to interview, or interview all eligible women. In either case, you would apply a sampling fraction to each village, such as one out of five households or one out of ten eligible women.

Nonprobability Sampling

Nonprobability sampling refers to the selection of a sample that is not based on known probabilities. It is distinguished from probability sampling by the fact that subjective judgments play a role in selecting the sampling elements.

Nonprobability sampling procedures are not valid for obtaining a sample that is truly representative of a larger population. Almost always, nonprobability samples tend to over-select some population elements and under-select others. When the known probabilities of selection are not known, there is no precise way to adjust for such distortions.

Despite these drawbacks, there are many instances in which obtaining a truly representative probability sample may be too difficult or too expensive. In fact, much, if not most, of HIV/AIDS operations research uses some kind of nonprobability sampling. For example, it is usually necessary to use nonprobability samples when studying sex workers and their clients, injecting drug users, and men who have sex with men. The external validity of intervention studies that use nonprobability sampling techniques depends on replication of the study results in different populations.

There are two broad types of nonprobability samples: (1) **convenience** samples, which are selected from whatever cases happen to be available at a given time or place, and (2) **purposive** samples, which consist of units deliberately selected to provide specific information about a population.

An example of a **convenience sample** in HIV/AIDS research might occur when you place an advertisement in a newspaper stating you want to interview men who have sex with men. The men who answered your advertisement would be a convenience sample. Similarly, if you wanted to find out how much condoms cost in pharmacies by visiting the five drugstores nearest to your office, you would be using a convenience sample.

A special type of convenience sample is the **snowball sample**. In this technique, persons who have agreed to be interviewed recommend acquaintances for interviewing. Your convenience sample of men answering an advertisement for men who have sex with men would become a snowball sample if you asked everyone who responded to the original advertisement to recruit other men who had sex with men for your study. It should be noted that internal validity is not compromised in a study that uses a nonprobability sample and then randomly assigns cases to an experimental and control group. However, external validity is compromised. The number of groups for which the results can be considered valid will be smaller than if a probability sample were used. In operations research some studies emphasize internal validity; others emphasize external validity or representativeness. Few are able to emphasize both internal and external validity.

Purposive samples are commonly used in qualitative and experimental operations research studies. If you conduct a focus group to select a name for a condom brand that is especially appealing to adolescent males, you might purposively include in your group only 15- to 19-year-old men. If the brand were to be marketed only in urban pharmacies, the sample might be further restricted to adolescent males who live in urban areas and have purchased a condom in a pharmacy in the past six months. When you conduct experiments, the costs and procedures needed to ensure internal validity often preclude use of a representative sample of the population. In selecting samples to include in an experiment, you might use a convenience sample (for example, a few clinics that volunteer to participate in the study), or, more often, you might purposively select units because they are either **critical cases** or **typical cases**.

A Ministry of Health might want to determine whether multipurpose, rural community health workers are capable of using the "syndromic" approach to diagnose and treat STIs in men. You might choose a group of health workers whom you think might have difficulty in implementing the new activity (perhaps because of limited literacy or the pressure of other activities). You might make this choice because you reason that if the weakest group of health workers can perform the task successfully, then average and above-average workers will also be able to perform it. Conversely, you might select a group of the most able community health workers to test your intervention, because you believe that if they are unable to implement the intervention successfully, all other community health workers will also be unable to implement the intervention. Either strategy would involve the selection of critical cases. If you wanted to draw a purposive sample of critical cases, you might select a group of workers whose educational level is within the modal range for the entire population of community health workers. The homogeneity in this sample would allow you to draw conclusions about whether or not the "typical worker" would experience problems implementing the intervention.

In contrast to the critical case or typical case approaches, you might want to draw a purposive sample that is somewhat representative of the heterogeneity found among community health workers. This type of sample is called a **quota sample**. In quota sampling you purposively select elements for your sample. There are two broad reasons for quota sampling:

- To ensure that the sample composition is proportionate to the population for variables believed critical to the study. In the case of the health worker experiment, you might draw a sample for which the educational distribution and distribution of years of experience of the workers are the same as for the population of community health workers.

- To obtain a desired sample size. For example, you might decide to visit all patients going to an STI clinic until you have interviews from 400 women and 400 men.

Sample Sizes

Many handbooks contain formulas for estimating sample size because the size of the sample is one of the most important determinants of the accuracy of survey estimates. However, we will not provide formulas for sample size estimation. Formulas differ among sampling strategies (for example, those used in cluster sampling are different from those used in simple random sampling); population size; the type of variable being studied; experimental design, if any; and type of statistical comparison planned. Explaining all of these formulas is beyond the scope of this *Handbook*, and presenting any single formula would be of little relevance to most OR studies. Rather, in the remainder of this chapter we will discuss some of the basic factors that affect sample size, to familiarize the reader with the concepts necessary to work with a sampler or select an appropriate formula from any standard textbook on sampling.

We will begin our discussion of sample size estimation with an important caveat. If your objective is to obtain a probability sample that is representative of a relatively large population, such as in a typical descriptive survey, you need to obtain the assistance of a sampling specialist. A nationally representative health survey may have sample sizes of 5,000 to 6,000 or more individuals. Sample sizes of this magnitude will allow accurate estimates of several different variables for different subpopulations, but the cost may be hundreds of thousands of dollars.

A sample size appropriate to the needs of a researcher depends on two concepts: **precision** and **confidence level**. Precision is the amount of sampling error that can be tolerated by the researcher. Confidence is the level of certainty that the true value of the variable being studied is captured within the **standard error**, or sampling error. A standard error is simply the difference between the true value of the variable in the population and the estimated value of the variable obtained from the sample.

In calculating sample size, the researcher and program decision maker must first decide how much precision they need in their estimate and how much confidence they need in the result. The greater the precision and confidence required, the larger the sample size needed. For some purposes, an error of ±10 percent might be tolerable, but for other purposes a standard error greater than 1 percent might not be tolerable. Usually, the degree of precision needed depends on the consequences of accepting a study finding as true when in fact it is not true—in other words, it is an error. If people may die because of an error, a great deal of precision is needed in the estimate. However, if the practical effects of an error are likely to be trivial and easily fixed, less precision may be acceptable.

Another important factor in determining sample size is the amount of resources available for the study. Do you have the resources for your study to afford a 1 percent error, or must you settle for a 5 percent error? While most people would prefer small errors, that requires large samples which, in turn, require large resources. The availability of resources usually determines the upper limit of the sample size used in surveys.

In discussing with a statistician or sample expert how large a sample you will need for your study, it is important to have a fairly good understanding of several key concepts, some of which have been introduced above. One of these concepts is the **standard error**.

The standard error is expressed as a range around a point estimate of a variable in a study. Suppose you interviewed a sample of 200 peer educators and found that 40 percent (the point estimate) had talked to someone about HIV/AIDS that day. It is quite unlikely that exactly 40 percent of your universe of peer educators talked about HIV/AIDS on the day of the interview. It is more likely that the true number is slightly different than your point estimate, by, say, plus or minus 3 percent. The interval extends above and below your point estimate (in this case 40 percent) because half the time the true population value will be below your point estimate, and half the time it will be above your point estimate. Thus, given an error of ± 3 percent, you would say that the number of all peer educators talking about HIV/AIDS on that day is between 37 and 43 percent. If you want greater precision, you need to have a smaller sampling error and therefore a larger sample size. A sample that captures the true population value within ± 3 percent provides a considerably more precise estimate than a sample that captures the true value within an interval of ±10 percent.

What is somewhat confusing is that this standard error interval is referred to as a **confidence interval**. In contrast, the **confidence level** is the degree of certainty (expressed as a probability) that the researcher has that the true population variable is captured within the confidence interval. Thus, in reporting the result of a survey of HIV prevalence, the researcher might say something like, "The survey estimates HIV prevalence in this region at 15.6 percent. We are 95 percent certain that true regional prevalence is between 13.6 and 17.6

percent," or more simply, "We can state with 95 percent confidence that HIV prevalence is 15.6 percent, plus or minus 3 percent."

So far, we have discussed sample size as a way of influencing the precision of an estimate of a single variable or observation. But in operations research intervention studies, researchers are usually interested in comparing two or more observations.

For example, you might ask: Has the proportion of sex workers who used a condom with their last client increased over time? Is the observed difference in increased condom use the result of your educational campaign or is it just due to sampling error? Is the difference between HIV/AIDS knowledge scores of experimental and control groups due to your new teaching approach or is it just chance?

OR studies should determine the sample size needed to detect real differences between variables during the project design phase by using an appropriate sample size formula. These formulas all require minimum information that the researcher must be able to provide the sampler, including the following:

- **The baseline value of the dependent variable.** For example, is the baseline value 10 percent prevalence, $12 per case treated, or 200 visits per month?

- **The size of the difference between two estimates that you want to find statistically significant.** The smaller the difference between the two estimates, the larger the sample needed. The reason for this is that standard errors must be smaller to detect a small difference than a large difference. For example, attributing a 1 percent change (for example, from 2 to 3 percent) in condom use to an intervention rather than to sampling error implies the need for a confidence interval around each point estimate that is less than ± 0.5 percent (the upper bound of your confidence interval around 2 percent is 2.5 percent; the lower bound of your confidence interval around 3 percent is also 2.5 percent). However, you need a much smaller sample size if you want to attribute a 50 percent difference (for example, from 20 to 30 percent) in condom use to your intervention rather than to sampling error. The confidence intervals only need to be less than ± 20 percent.

- **The significance level.** This refers to the probability that the size of the observed difference between the two variables could have been produced by sampling error or by chance rather than by the intervention. The smaller the significance level, the lower the probability that the result could be the result of chance. Thus, a significance level of .1 means that the probability that the observed difference was produced by chance is 1 in 10. A significance level of .01 means that the probability that the difference was produced by chance is 1 in 100. Traditionally, significance levels are usually set at .05 (or 1 chance in 20). The smaller the probability of finding a difference that is the result of chance or sampling error, the larger the sample size required. Thus, to reduce the probability that the result is due to chance from 1 in 20 to 1 in 100 can, for a given difference, increase required sample sizes from 70 to 90 percent.

- **The confidence level.** This is the probability that the true value is within the specified confidence interval (see above).

Usually, other issues also need to be addressed in the sample size formula. If a cluster sample will be used, it is necessary to adjust sample size upward. If the sample is from a small universe (less than 10,000 units), a multiplier (the finite population correction) can be used to adjust sample size downward.

What To Do: Sampling

1. Decide first whether you want to draw a sample and, if so, whether it should be a probability sample or a nonprobability sample. In making this decision, take into account the objectives of the study, the extent to which the findings need to be representative of a larger population, and such resource factors as cost, time, and personnel.

2. Calculate the size of the sample required for your study. Seek the assistance of a statistician to do this, if possible. The statistician needs to know your estimates of the values of the variables to be tested, the degree of accuracy needed, and so on. It is always better to have a somewhat larger sample than required instead of a smaller one to conduct the research.

CHAPTER 9

DATA COLLECTION

Discussion of how data will be collected is an important part of the methodological section of your proposal. There are many different ways to collect data. The approach you choose depends on the study objectives, the study design, and the availability of time, money, and personnel. In deciding on the best way to collect data, it is important to consider whether the study is intended to produce **quantitative**, numerical findings or to produce **qualitative**, descriptive information.

Most operations research studies are concerned with the quantitative measurement of program operations, but many also are (or should be) concerned with detailed qualitative information on processes (for example, how a project is actually implemented in the field, how couples decide to use condoms, or how PLHA can become more involved in the implementation of programs). Often, study objectives call for both quantitative and qualitative information, which may require that you use more than one data collection method.

Quantitative Data

One of the most common ways to collect quantitative data on people is to use a standard questionnaire that is administered by a trained interviewer. There are other ways to collect quantitative data, including self-administered questionnaires, service statistics, or such secondary sources as the census, vital records, an HIV/AIDS sentinel surveillance system, or other existing records and reports.

If a study's sample is composed of geographic or organizational units (such as villages, districts, clinics, hospitals, and VCT centers) rather than people, quantitative data usually can be obtained from service statistics and secondary sources. If information is not available from such sources, it may be necessary to obtain data on geographic or organizational units by interviewing people who are members of these units or are knowledgeable about them.

Structured Interviews

Studies that obtain data by interviewing people are called **surveys**. If the people interviewed are a representative sample of a larger population, such studies are called **sample surveys**. If the sample is large enough to permit statistical analysis, it is customary to use structured interviews rather than unstructured ones, since the former lend themselves better to quantitative analysis and the latter create serious data processing difficulties, particularly if the sample is large.

A structured interview is one that uses a standard questionnaire (or interview schedule) to ensure that all respondents are asked exactly the same set of questions in the same sequence. The exact wording of each question is specified in advance, and the interviewer merely reads each question to the respondent. In designing a questionnaire and then using interviewers to administer it, you need to remember several points:

Use simple language that can be easily understood by the respondents.

Precode the responses to the questions whenever possible so that the information can be transferred easily to a computer and then tabulated. This requires more effort when designing the interview schedule, but the time saved during the processing and analysis more than compensate for it.

Try to avoid embarrassing or painful questions. If it is necessary to ask a sensitive question, word it as tactfully as possible and avoid asking it near the beginning of the interview, when the respondent is less relaxed. It is generally best to put sensitive questions in the middle of the questionnaire.

Don't use leading questions that strongly suggest a particular response. For example, in a survey of sex workers, the following would be a leading question: "Most sex workers in the world experience violence from their clients. Have you also experienced violence from your clients?"

Avoid asking for more than one item of information in a single question. For instance, do not ask, "Do you and your husband want another child?" If the respondent and her husband disagree about having another child, an answer of either "yes" or "no" will be impossible to interpret accurately. A response of "yes" could mean "I want another child," "My husband wants a child," or "Both of us want a child." It would be better to ask two separate questions: "Do you want another child?" "Does your husband want another child?"

Watch out for ambiguous wording of questions. For instance, if you are conducting a survey among women, a question such as "Do you use a contraceptive when you have sex with your partner?" may seem clear enough. But since the respondents are women, some of them may answer "no" even though their partner has had a vasectomy or uses a condom; these are male methods used by men, not women. A better way to word the question would be to ask, "Do you or your partner use a contraceptive when you have sex?"

Do not overload your interview schedule with questions that are not essential for your study. Keep it as short as possible to avoid tiring your respondent and to simplify the data processing and analysis.

Include all questions necessary to provide sufficient information on the variables you want to study. Also be sure that the data necessary to test the hypotheses of the study can be obtained from the questionnaire instruments. It is often helpful to prepare a list of key study variables with an indication of where the data for each variable will be obtained. For example, to be sure that all variables in your study have a source of information, you should create the following type of table:

Variable	Source of Data
Age	Question 5
Attitude toward HIV/AIDS	Questions 8, 10, 26, 28, 32
HIV status	Sero laboratory test
Contact with peer educator	Questions 14 and 15
HIV prevalence district	Sentinel surveillance

Start with the easier questions, and move on to the ones that are more sensitive or difficult after the respondent has had an opportunity to become accustomed to the interview situation. Respondents are likely to be somewhat tense or even suspicious at the beginning of the interview, so a major task of the interviewer during the first few minutes is to establish rapport in order to put the respondent at ease. This task is easier if the initial questions are not likely to cause embarrassment or be difficult to answer.

Ask all respondents each question in exactly the same way. If the interview is to be conducted in more than one language, prepare full written translations in all major languages and instruct your interviewers to use those translations word for word. Do not permit free translations, except for languages with too few respondents to justify the cost of preparing written translations. To ensure comparability of wording among the various written translations, have them "**back-translated**" into the original language to verify that the meaning is retained. The back translation should be done by persons who are not familiar with the original wording of the questionnaire.

Pretest the questionnaire in an actual field situation. Here are several principles of pretesting that should be noted:

1. The pretest does not need to involve large numbers of respondents; 30–50 respondents are often enough if they are sampled (purposively) in a way that ensures that the expected heterogeneity of the study sample is reflected in the pretest sample. This means making sure that the pretest includes the same types of respondents who will be included in the study sample: old and young, urban and rural, less educated and more educated, males and females, and so on.

2. Be prepared to conduct more than one pretest. If a pretest results in major revisions, it is a good idea to conduct a second pretest to be sure the revisions are satisfactory.

3. Pretesting should be completed before the training of interviewers. Often it is possible to use field supervisors to do the pretest. This gives them a clearer understanding of study objectives and better prepares them to help train the interviewers.

4. The main purpose of the pretest is to ensure that the respondents are able to understand the questions and answer them usefully. Hence, it is not enough simply to interview the pretest respondents; rather, each interview should be followed by a **debriefing**. During the debriefing the interviewer asks about the respondent's understanding of questions that are likely to be misunderstood or that appear to have caused difficulty during the interview.

Provide complete training for all interviewers.
The training should be designed to familiarize the interviewers with the intent and meaning of the questions, let them role-play interview situations, and give them experience in actually conducting interviews in the field under supervision. Provide them with an instruction manual that clearly explains procedures for completing questionnaires. Be sure the training is of sufficient duration for the trainees to become skilled at interviewing. One of the most serious mistakes that can be made by a study investigator is to provide inadequate training to interviewers.

An appointment should be made for an interview callback if a prospective respondent is not available during the interviewer's first visit. It is common to require at least two callbacks before dismissing a sample case as unavailable for interview.

Interviewers must be given clear instructions for obtaining substitutes. If a study sample is small, it may be necessary to find substitutes for cases that cannot be located. Interviewers need to know how to select substitute cases that will ensure either a random sampling of substitutes or a selection of substitutes who are similar to the cases originally selected. However, if the sample is large enough to tolerate some loss of cases, it is usually better not to use substitutes.

Isolate the respondent during the interview. If other people are present, the respondent's answers may be influenced by them. For example, if a man is interviewed in the presence of his wife, he may not be entirely honest in replying to a question about the number of casual partners he has had sex with in the last month.

Check all completed interview schedules for errors, omissions, and discrepancies as soon after interviewing as possible. Respondents should be revisited to correct errors that cannot be otherwise

resolved. It is best to have the interviewer check the questionnaire immediately after the interview so that the respondent can be consulted. After the interviewer has checked and corrected the questionnaire, it should be rechecked by the field supervisor. This checking process is known as **field editing**.

Service Statistics

All national HIV/AIDS control and coordinating organizations generate program statistics, as do many service delivery organizations. Some organizations have established a management information system (MIS). The quality of service statistics, however, varies from country to country and even within countries and thus these statistics should be used with caution.

Service statistics often help researchers define the parameters of the problem they want to study. In some cases, service statistics can be used to compare the results of a particular study with nationwide figures. In operations research projects it is often necessary to design supplementary forms to provide data that are not available from the regular service statistics.

Service statistics have the advantage of being an inexpensive data source. Using service statistics instead of surveys can save many thousands of dollars in research costs. However, the type of data available is more limited than data obtained from a survey, and service statistics data often have serious reliability problems. Two common problems are that they are often incomplete and that providers are not trained to correctly fill in the forms. Before doing a study that relies on service statistics, be sure to assess the reliability of the data.

Self-administered Questionnaires

If money, personnel, and time allow, interviews are generally preferable to self-administered questionnaires. For most surveys in developing countries, self-administered questionnaires are difficult if not impossible to use because many respondents are not educated enough to complete questionnaires themselves.

There are other problems with self-administered questionnaires, even among educated respondents:

- Instructions or questions are more likely to be misunderstood without an interviewer to help explain them.
- Portions of the questionnaire are more likely to be left blank.
- It is difficult to incorporate many conditional sequences of questions (for example, "If the response to question 12 is 'yes,' go to question 13; if not, skip to question 18") without causing confusion.

Self-administered questionnaires are likely to be useful in situations where literate respondents are already gathered together in a setting where they can, for example, write in a classroom or an office. Self-administered questionnaires can be especially useful in evaluating school-based HIV/AIDS programs or training programs for peer educators. They may also produce more accurate results on such sensitive topics as sexual behavior.

Sometimes, blank questionnaires are mailed out to respondents, who are asked to complete them and send them back. This method has the virtue of being very inexpensive but also has all the drawbacks noted above, plus the added problem of high nonresponse rates. It is common for mailed questionnaires to elicit less than a 10 to 20 percent return, even after one or two reminders. This drawback affects how representative the sample is and may render the validity of quantitative findings so questionable that they are of very little use.

Situation Analysis

An approach that has been used in recent years to collect information on the functioning of an entire service delivery system is called a **Situation Analysis**. This approach can be used to examine, for example, how prepared the formal health care system of a country is to address the needs of HIV/AIDS clients.

The Situation Analysis approach involves visiting a relatively large number of randomly selected service delivery points (SDPs), usually clinics or hospitals; interviewing managers, providers, and clients at these SDPs, using structured interviews; conducting a full inventory of the SDP's equipment and commodities on the day of the visit; and observing the client-provider interaction at the SDPs on the day of the visit. This methodology allows you to collect a relatively large and detailed amount of information on the functioning of the health care system and the type and quality of HIV/AIDS services that are available. A limiting factor is that when a large number of SDPs are sampled, the cost of conducting a Situation Analysis study can be high.

Secondary Data Sources

Information from recent censuses, vital statistics, sentinel surveillance systems, UNAIDS, WHO, ILO, the World Bank, and even previous surveys can often be used with data collected especially for a study to enrich the analysis. A large body of data on health and HIV/AIDS has been collected by many organizations and by national surveys such as the Demographic and Health Surveys. Much of this information is available through the internet (see the list of internet addresses in the bibliography).

Content Analysis of Written Materials

This method is usually not used as the sole method in an HIV/AIDS operations research study, but it can serve as a useful adjunct to other types of data collection and analysis. For instance, the content of documents related to a training curriculum may be analyzed to determine what type of knowledge and skills the training is supposed to develop. The content analysis can guide the researcher in devising procedures to test the knowledge and skills of the trainees.

Information and education materials on HIV/AIDS can be "content analyzed" to indicate whether messages are being overemphasized or underemphasized. The content of press reports or public statements made by policymakers can be studied to assess attitudes toward HIV/AIDS and issues concerning HIV/AIDS stigma and discrimination. Research reports may also be content analyzed to determine the current state of knowledge about a particular research topic.

Qualitative Data

The data collection techniques most appropriate for studies whose objectives call for descriptive, qualitative data tend to be different from those most appropriate for quantitative analysis. Operations research studies often use a combination of quantitative and qualitative data collection methods to obtain the most accurate and realistic picture of a program situation. Quantitative methods discussed earlier are important for obtaining data for making predictions, "probabilistic" statements, and generalizations. Qualitative methods such as unstructured interviews, focus group discussions, and direct observation of operations are important to obtain data on processes, on how and why a program works, and on unintended and unanticipated program outcomes.

Unstructured Interviews

The chief drawback of structured interviews is that the responses obtained tend to be short and sometimes superficial. An alternative approach to interviewing, which permits greater depth of meaning, is to seek detailed, open-ended responses to questions. Such interviews are often called **in-depth interviews**. Instead of reading formal questions from a structured interview schedule, the interviewer has an outline of topics or a set of general questions to serve as a guide to the kind of information required. Details that are not brought out initially are sought through follow-up questions called **probes**.

The chief drawbacks of unstructured interviews are that (1) the interviews require highly skilled and experienced interviewers, and (2) the analysis can be complex and time-consuming. The shortage of qualified interviewers and analysts and the high cost of conducting and processing such interviews usually mean that a small sample size must be used (sometimes as few as 20–30 respondents).

In-depth interviews are usually most useful in exploratory studies that seek to clarify concepts or generate hypotheses before developing questionnaires for quantitative surveys. They also are useful for generating supplementary, explanatory data to augment the findings from larger surveys. For example, little is known about the gender and power dynamics involved in the negotiation between sex workers and their clients regarding the use of condoms. An unstructured interview could help gain insight into the dynamics and determinants of the decision to use or not to use condoms.

Focus Group Discussion

A way of reducing the amount of time and number of personnel required for conducting and analyzing in-depth interviews is to bring respondents together in discussion groups that focus on a particular topic. The use of **focus group** discussions has the advantage of being economical yet still yields detailed qualitative information from a relatively large number of respondents. It is often an excellent technique to use for examining group or community consensus about a particular issue.

The interviewer (or facilitator) follows nearly the same procedure as in unstructured interviews, using a general discussion guide and eliciting details through probes. Participants are usually sampled purposively to reflect population variations that are particularly relevant to the research topic. For instance, cases sampled for focus group discussions might consist of a group of truck drivers, adolescents, sex workers, teachers, or another group of interest. While focus group discussions can generate extremely valuable information, they are not easy to conduct. To obtain meaningful information, a highly skilled and trained facilitator must guide the group but not lead it in a predetermined direction. Also, the analysis of transcripts from focus group discussions is not easy; if not done correctly, this can sometimes generate findings that are more fiction than fact.

Direct Observation of Operations

This technique can generate either quantitative or qualitative data, but tends to be used more for small-scale exploratory studies than for large-scale quantitative studies. The reason for this is that it usually requires relatively highly skilled observers and analysts and prolonged periods of observation, resulting in a high cost per unit of observation. This technique lends itself particularly well to observation of community responses to program efforts. It is the chief method of ethnographers, who specialize in community studies. It is also useful for organizational studies, such as observation of clinic operations, activities of field workers, and administrative procedures. The researcher should note, however, that when workers are being observed they often do not behave in ways that are typical of their day-to-day behavior.

What To Do: Data Collection

1. Review your study objectives and hypotheses as well as your list of independent and dependent variables. What types of information do you require? Which data gathering technique(s) would be most appropriate and feasible for gathering the desired information? Is some of the information already available from other sources?

2. If you intend to collect information through a survey, review the list of points under the heading Structured Interviews. Be sure your proposal discusses important steps, such as translation, pretesting, training of interviewers, and rules about callbacks and substitutions.

3. Make an outline of the data gathering instrument(s) you intend to use (for example, the interview schedule, discussion guide, or observation guide). Give examples in the proposal of questions to be asked, especially those designed to elicit information about key variables found in the hypotheses. Be sure you incorporate measures (or at least descriptions of measures) of all the variables you intend to study. It is useful to list all the variables of the study and then under each variable record the question or questions that will be used in the questionnaire. Here are some examples:

   Variable 1: Condom use
   - Q1: Have you ever used a condom?
   - Q2: Did you use a condom the last time you had sex?
   - Q3: Do you use a condom with casual partners?

   Variable 2: Education
   - Q4: What is the highest grade in school you have completed?

4. Describe your data collection procedures and include the description with the outline of the data gathering instrument(s) in the proposal.

Data Quality Checks

There are several ways to check the quality of interview data:

- Sometimes a researcher will deliberately ask two or more questions that yield the same type of information. The first question might be asked at the beginning of the interview and the second at the end. The two questions are then examined for consistency of response. This is one way to check the reliability of the data.
- For difficult questions, sensitive questions, or questions for which the researchers want to be sure the information is correct, the interviewers can be instructed to probe. That is, the interviewer can repeat the question in a slightly different form or repeat the respondent's answer and then ask if the information is correct. For example, a woman might report that she has two sons and three daughters. The interviewer might then say, "You have a total of five children, two males and three females. Is that correct? Are there any other children you may have forgotten to tell me about?"
- Field supervisors should be used to help the interviewers with difficult situations and to make sure that they are actually doing their work. (Occasionally, interviewers complete their questionnaires in tea stalls or beer halls!) Some studies use a ratio of one supervisor for every five interviewers.
- For most studies using an interview procedure, an attempt is made to re-interview a certain percentage of the respondents. Depending on the size of the sample, a general rule is to re-interview between 5 and 10 percent of the sample. The data from the first interview are then checked against the data from the second interview for consistency. This is another check on the reliability of the data. Obviously, if there are major inconsistencies, particularly on such demographic profile questions as age, marital status, and parity, there is a problem somewhere. The problem might be with the questionnaire, the interviewers, the tabulation procedures, or something else.
- Once the data have been collected and tabulated, it is possible to do statistical checks for errors or for consistency of response. For example, a frequency distribution of the parity of women may reveal that several women claim to have 18 or 19 living children. Since this is highly unlikely, the investigator is faced with the choice of either discarding the entire questionnaire, eliminating at least the information from the question on parity, or going back and re-interviewing the women who claim to have 18 or 19 children.

What To Do: Data Quality Checks

Describe the procedures you will use to check the quality of the data collected. Consider the following procedures:

1. Include repeat questions in your questionnaire that can be used to check for consistency of response.

2. Have supervisors monitor the work of the interviewers in the field.

3. Re-interview a percentage of respondents and look for inconsistencies.

4. Recode a percentage of the questionnaires to be sure that there are no coding errors.

5. Examine the frequency distribution on all variables to see if there are odd codes or items that are not logical.

Confidentiality of Information

It is always important to maintain the confidentiality of the information collected from respondents. Unless absolutely required, do not collect information that is sensitive or potentially harmful. Whenever possible, use code numbers instead of names. Assure the respondents that the information they give will be kept confidential. Do not let other people use the information you have collected when there is a chance that the use of the information could be damaging to the respondent. You have an obligation to protect the confidentiality of the respondents in your study.

Operations research on the topic of HIV/AIDS often involves asking very sensitive questions and collecting information that, if disclosed, might create problems for the respondent. Questionnaires should always be stored in a closed, locked cabinet. During the training of interviewers and supervisors, it is extremely important to thoroughly cover the topic of confidentiality and informed consent. If respondents do not want to be interviewed, you have an obligation to respect their wishes. Use an **informed consent form** to explain the basic nature of the study and obtain the agreement of the respondent to be interviewed. The informed consent form should be written in simple, plain language that is understandable to everyone. During data collection, it is important to make spot checks to be sure that the informed consent form is being used by the interviewers.

What To Do: Confidentiality of Information

1. Describe in detail how you plan to maintain
    the confidentiality of information collected,
    including how you are going to store question-
    naires and use code numbers instead of names.

2. Describe the training process you will use to
    instruct interviewers and supervisors on the use
    of the informed consent form.

3. Include a sample of the informed consent form
    in your study proposal.

CHAPTER 10

TABULATION OF DATA

In your proposal, you should discuss editing and tabulating data immediately after data collection procedures. Although qualitative methods are being increasingly used in operations research, most OR studies still involve quantitative analysis that requires statistical manipulation of the information collected.

First, you need to convert the information into a form that will allow it to be analyzed. Second, you must specify the statistical manipulations to be performed. Finally, you need to present the important findings resulting from these manipulations in a report or series of reports.

Preparing Tabulations

Any recently produced desktop computer probably has the hardware capability needed to process an operations research data set. However, unless the computer you use is located at a research organization or a health program evaluation unit, it may not have the software needed for statistical analysis. This is not a problem when data consist only of service statistics from a small number of service delivery points, or when modeling or conducting a cost analysis; in both cases, spreadsheets are adequate for analyzing OR data. However, it's more likely that you will need to perform many statistical tests, analyze survey data, or work with a very large data set and will need more powerful statistical software.

Epi Info is a statistical package that is available free of charge from the U.S. Centers for Disease Control and Prevention (CDC). It has features for processing and analyzing data, including survey data. Although it is a basic package, it has all the features necessary for analyzing most OR studies. More powerful (and expensive) software packages include *SPSS, STATA,* and *SAS,* all of which require training to use. In deciding on software, it is wise to select a program that is widely used in your country or in your organization, since it will then be much easier to find technical support and consultants.

Data Coding

All statistical packages include data entry features. But before you begin to enter data, you must transform the raw information for tabulation and analysis. Nonnumerical data that are to be analyzed quantitatively must be converted into numerical codes. If your data gathering instrument uses mainly closed questions (a question with a limited number of possible predetermined responses, such as "yes" or "no"), the best approach is to **precode** the instrument. Thus, the question would appear with the numeric codes for the responses already printed on the instrument, as shown in the example below:

Question No.	Question	Response	Skip To
110	Where did you get your HIV test?	Hope Hospital = 1 Central Hospital = 2 Town Clinic = 3 Military Camp = 4 Other (Specify) Nonresponse = 9	→ Q115 → Q116 → Q117

If, in response to question 110, the respondent states that he received his last HIV test at Central Hospital, the interviewer would circle the number 2. If the answer is the military camp, the interviewer would circle 4. Before beginning computerized data entry, you should check all questionnaires to make sure that the interviewers have recorded a response to each question.

If the number of categories for a particular variable (including, if relevant, codes for "nonresponse," "not applicable," "don't know," and "other") is less than 10, numerical codes should be single-digit numerals. If the total possible number of categories is between 10 and 99, two-digit codes should be used instead. For some variables, it may be necessary to use three-digit, four-digit, or even larger codes; for example, calendar dates typically require four or more digits.

Data Entry and Editing

Coded data need to be entered into the computer with a minimum of typing errors and then edited to correct any errors in the data. In entering data, the researcher should use the data verification procedures available with most statistical packages. In verification, the same data are entered twice. The verification program indicates discrepancies in the numbers entered. In the example above, the first data entry clerk might have entered the number 3. However, the second time the response is entered, it may be entered as 1. When such discrepancies occur, the program signals the data entry person to check the data entry form for the correct number.

In addition to verification, the researcher should check for the following types of errors:

- **"Ilegal" codes:** Values that are not specified in the coding instructions. For example, a code of "7" in question 110 above would be an illegal code. The best way to check for illegal codes is to have the computer produce a frequency distribution and check it for illegal codes.

- **Omissions:** For example, a failure by an interviewer to follow correctly the SKIP instructions in a questionnaire. This would be the case in question 110, if the interviewer failed to skip to question 115 after a response of "Central Hospital."

- **Logical inconsistencies:** For example, a respondent whose current age is less than her age at marriage.

- **Improbabilities:** For example, a 25-year-old woman with ten living children.

Once you find errors, check the original data forms to make the necessary corrections. Most coded data can be edited on the computer, but **field editing** should always be done by supervisors whenever there is a chance that the error can be corrected by talking with the data gatherer or perhaps re-interviewing the respondent for clarification.

Variable Transformations

Once data have been entered into the database, it is often necessary to transform variables. The transformations may constitute the entire analysis of the study, but far more often data transformations are done to permit subsequent analyses.

For instance, instead of having the questionnaire record the respondent's age, the questionnaire may record only the month and year of birth. If age is a variable to be studied, it can be obtained simply by having the computer subtract the month and year of birth from the month and year of the interview.

This transformed variable might be transformed even further for certain kinds of additional analysis. For example, if you want to cross-tabulate age by other variables, it is preferable to limit the age distribution to relatively few age categories (usually five- or ten-year categories) or even to dichotomize (for example, ages 15–29 and ages 30 or more). You can use several methods to transform variables, the most common of which are listed below.

RECODES

In recoding, category labels are changed. This technique is used to "collapse" large numbers of variable categories into smaller numbers. For example, single years of age can be collapsed and transformed into age categories, such as ages 15–19, 20–24, and 25–29.

COUNTS

If you are collecting information on whether the respondents have ever used any of eight services for persons with HIV/AIDS, you might want to count the number of services ever used by each respondent. Thus, you could generate a new variable that might be called "Number of Services Ever Used."

CONDITIONAL TRANSFORMATIONS

When the nature of the transformation of one variable depends on the second variable, conditional transformations may be useful. For instance, suppose you asked respondents three questions:

- Did you hear the partner reduction radio message in July?
- How many casual sex partners did you have between April and June?
- How many casual sex partners did you have between August and October?

With the information from these three questions, you could then create a new variable called "Partner Reduction among Persons Exposed to Radio Message." This can be done by subtracting the number of partners in question 3 from the number in question 2. But you would do this only if the answer to question one is "yes."

OTHER MATHEMATICAL TRANSFORMATIONS

Calculating age from the date of birth and the date of the interview is an example of a mathematical transformation. Another example is obtaining an HIV prevalence rate by dividing the number of HIV-positive individuals in a community by the number of residents.

What To Do: Coding and Editing

1. Be sure to check the availability of computers, statistical packages, and programming assistance before you start.

2. Indicate in the proposal the checking and editing that you will do.

3. Precode your questionnaire or other instrument.

4. Prepare a codebook that labels and specifies the meaning of each numerical value of all variables in your database.

5. Plan for editing during field work.

6. Verify the accuracy of the numerical values entered into the database.

7. When data entry has been completed, check for illegal codes, omissions, inconsistencies, and improbabilities before analyzing your data.

8. Begin to perform basic variable transformations.

CHAPTER 11

DATA ANALYSIS

Plan for Data Analysis

One of the most important parts of an OR proposal is the plan for data analysis. Although the data analysis plan is usually located near the end of a proposal, you must know which analyses you plan to perform early in the design phase of any study. A cardinal rule is to never design a study without first knowing how you plan to analyze the data.

You need to indicate in your proposal which analytical approaches are most appropriate for meeting your study objectives. A prime consideration in selecting an analytical procedure is the extent to which it is appropriate for answering your research questions. Another important factor to keep in mind is how well you or someone associated with the data processing and analysis understands the terms and operations involved in the analytical procedure chosen and how well that person can interpret the results correctly. All statistical tests and measures referred to below are widely used by social scientists.

This section will introduce you to the names of these procedures, help you understand when it is permissible to use them, and explain in as nontechnical a way as possible the underlying principles for the tests most frequently used in HIV/AIDS operations research. No formulas are given and no data manipulations required by the tests are explained. A handbook such as this one cannot make you an expert in statistics or in data analysis. For the researcher or manager who wants to learn how to calculate and interpret the procedures discussed in this section, we recommend almost any introductory textbook on statistical methods. In addition, you can consult a number of very helpful internet addresses that explain the use of various statistical procedures (some of these are listed in the appendices).

Analytic Procedures I

Attributes of the Data

The purpose of data analysis is to provide answers to the research questions being studied. The research question also dictates the type of data to be collected during a study and the type of analyses to be performed. For almost all studies, we want to describe what is typical of the group studied and how the cases differ from each other. Our measure of what is typical is called the **central tendency**. Our measure of how the cases differ is called the **variance or dispersion** in the data.

CENTRAL TENDENCY OR CHARACTERISTIC OF THE DATA
Once data have been cleaned and entered and any necessary transformations performed, you are ready to begin analysis.

In doing OR studies, you usually want to compare measures of central tendency. A researcher may want to compare the **mean** HIV/AIDS knowledge score of a group of students who saw a one-hour film on HIV/AIDS with a group of students who were given three one-hour lectures. Similarly,

before assigning clinics to treatment and control groups for a VCT intervention, the researcher may want to match the clinics on **median** client income. In writing a report on the activities of a social marketing project, a consultant might want to mention the most frequently charged, or **modal**, price of a brand of condoms.

The mean, the median, and the mode are measures of central tendency. The mean is simply an arithmetic average. It is the sum of individual scores divided by the number of individuals. The median is the midpoint measure in a group of measures: Half of the observations fall above the median and half below. The mode is the most frequently occurring figure in a set of figures. Each of these statistical measures describes the typical characteristic or tendency of a group in a slightly different way.

VARIANCE IN THE DATA
Often a researcher is interested not only in the average characteristic of a group but also in the variance or dispersion within the group, that is, how individuals in a group differ from the average or central tendency of the group. For example, if the mean age of first voluntary HIV testing is 28, what is the **range** in ages of the group? What are the ages of the youngest person tested and the oldest person tested? A group with a mean of 28 years but with a range of 24 to 30 years at first testing is probably quite different from another group with a mean of 28 years but with ages at first testing that range from 15 to 59.

The term **variance** is used when researchers measure dispersion around a **mean**. A common statistical measure of variation within a group is the **standard deviation**. This measure gives the average distance of individual measurement observations from the group mean. The larger the standard deviation, the greater the variation in the individual observations. The formulas of some commonly used statistical tests of differences between means such as the t test and the F test, also called the analysis of variance (ANOVA), use variance estimates to establish whether differences are statistically significant.

Other Measures of Dispersion

You can obtain other measures of dispersion in the data by counting the number of cases in each category. The resulting count is called a **frequency distribution**.

Occasionally researchers are interested in no further statistical manipulations of the data than the frequency distribution itself. For example, if you wanted to check the accuracy of a clinic director's statement that "the clinic is used by persons of all ages," you might do a frequency distribution of ages or examine the age distribution of clients. But more often you will want to go beyond such simple measurements. The nature of the statistical manipulations that are possible depends on the type of variable or, more accurately, on the level of measurement.

Before examining the central tendency and variance of data, you must first decide on the type of measurement that you will use. For example, is it more appropriate to use a median or a mean? Can you calculate the variance in the data? The type of analytic procedure or measurement that you can apply to a variable depends on the characteristics of the variable.

Classification of Variables

Earlier in this *Handbook* we discussed independent and dependent variables. Although variables can be characterized in many ways, for the purposes of data analysis we classify variables by a **measurement scale**. A scale is a rule for assigning numbers to objects or events. The type of scale that characterizes a variable also determines the types of analyses or measurements that can or cannot be performed on that variable. There are four levels of variable measurement: **nominal, ordinal, interval,** and **ratio**.

NOMINAL MEASUREMENT SCALES

In nominal measurements, the categories of variables differ from one another **in name only**. In other words, one category of a variable is not necessarily higher or lower, or greater or smaller than another category; it is just different in name.

For example, the variable sexual orientation has three categories: heterosexual, homosexual, and bisexual. A researcher could assign the number 1 to the category heterosexual, and 2 to homosexual, and 3 to bisexual. The only meaning these numbers have is to distinguish one category from the other. The researcher could just as well assign the number 3 to the category heterosexual, 1 to homosexual, and 2 to bisexual; it makes no difference. The only important consideration is to consistently use the same number for the same category. A special type of nominal variable is a **dichotomous variable**, which can take only one of two values. Examples of dichotomous variables include seropositive status (positive or negative) or sex (male or female).

Only very limited statistical manipulations are possible with nominal variables. In examining central tendency, you can calculate the mode (the most frequently occurring number). In looking at dispersion, you can calculate a percentage or frequency distribution. But you cannot calculate a mean or a standard deviation. It makes no sense to speak of the "mean sexually transmitted disease," or the average distance from "female."

ORDINAL MEASUREMENT SCALES

When there is a "rank-ordered" relationship among the categories, the variable is said to be an **ordinal variable**. In other words, a category that is assigned the number 4 might be considered higher than a category assigned the number 3, which would be higher than the category assigned the number 2. For example, respondents might be asked about their attitude toward widespread condom advertising. The response categories might be assigned numbers in the following manner:

4 = Approve very much
3 = Approve somewhat
2 = Approve very little
1 = Do not approve at all

The numbers assigned to the categories not only distinguish whether things are in the same category or a different category (as they do with nominal variables), but also indicate an **ordered ranking** from 4, which equals high (approve very much), to 1, which equals low (do not approve at all).

With ordinal variables, you can use all the statistical manipulations appropriate for nominal variables (such as the mode and the frequency distribution). Because there is a rank order to the numbers, you can also use the median and the percentile. But you cannot use a mean, or a standard deviation. It makes no sense to speak about the mean attitude of respondents to condom advertising. The reason is that the distance or interval between the categories is not known.

In the example above, you do not know if the distance between 1 (approve very much) and 2 (approve somewhat) is the same as the distance between 3 (approve very little) and 4 (do not approve at all). It might be that respondents who fall into categories 1, 2, and 3 are really very similar to each other, while those who fall into category 4 are very different. You could represent this situation as shown in Figure 11.1. While there is a rank order in the numbers assigned to the categories of the variable, the distance between the categories is not equal.

FIGURE 11.1
Ordinal measurement of the attitude
toward the use of advertising to
promote condom use

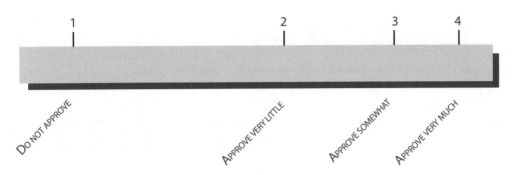

In HIV/AIDS operations research, ordinal variables are usually used to measure attitudes, beliefs, and opinions. Scale, in addition to referring to the type of measurements that can be used with a given type of data, has a second meaning. A scale can also be a group of related items that describe a response to a single variable. The items in a scale are arranged in order of importance or intensity, as in the example given above of the measurement of attitudes toward condom advertising.

The scale is constructed by presenting respondents with a statement followed by a series of response options indicating different degrees of agreement with the statement. Usually between three and ten response options are used in constructing these scales. Respondents are asked to indicate the option that most closely reflects their attitude or opinion. This type of scale is often referred to as a "**Likert Scale**," named after one of its originators, R. Likert.

INTERVAL MEASUREMENT SCALES
An **interval variable** is one in which the distance (or interval) between any two categories is known, is the same, and is constant. Interval variables have all the characteristics of nominal and ordinal variables plus the added characteristic of a constant unit of measurement between categories that are equally spaced.

Temperature and calendar dates are examples of interval variables. For example, the difference between the beginning of day 1 and the beginning of day 2 is 24 hours, just as it is between day 3 and day 4. With interval variables such as temperature, you can say that a temperature of 80 °F is 40 °F warmer than a temperature of 40 °F. However, an important point is that 80 °F cannot be said to be twice as warm as 40 ° because interval variables do not have a true zero point. At best, they have zero points that are set by convention or convenience.

The lack of a true zero point means that you cannot calculate ratios with interval data. However, you can calculate all of the measures of central tendency and dispersion that are allowed with nominal and ordinal variables plus the mean and and standard deviation. True interval variables are mainly encountered in the natural sciences and are not often found in OR studies. However, ratio variables, the fourth measurement level, are very frequently encountered in operations research.

RATIO MEASUREMENT SCALES
A **ratio scale** differs from an interval scale by having a **true zero point**. Age and number of living children are ratio variables, as are HIV incidence and prevalence, periods of time, number of clinic visits, and number of sexual partners. As is true for an interval scale, for a ratio scale it is possible to say that HIV incidence in one area is

FIGURE 11.2
Ratio measurement of number of sexual partners in last six months

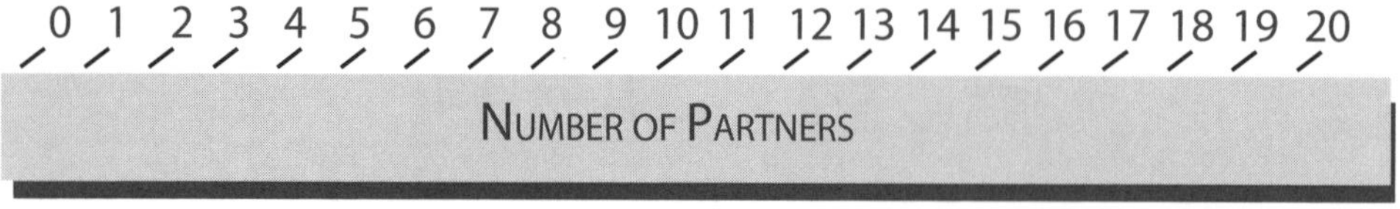

0 1 2 3 4 5 6 7 8 9 10 11 12 13 14 15 16 17 18 19 20

NUMBER OF PARTNERS

twice that in another, or that one clinic sees five times as many clients as another.

Figure 11.2 shows the number of sexual partners as a ratio scale. As is true for a nominal scale, you can say that someone with six sexual partners is different from someone with two sexual partners. As is true for an ordinal scale, you can say that a person with six partners has had more partners than someone with two partners. As is true for an interval scale, you can say that one person has had four more partners than another person. In addition, because you have a ratio scale with a true zero, you can also say that one person has had three times as many partners as the other.

As you can see, the characteristics of the four measurement scales are cumulative. All the statistics that you can use in analyzing nominal data can be used in analyzing ordinal data, plus you can use additional analyses that cannot be used with nominal data. Similarly, all the analyses that you can use with nominal, ordinal, and interval data can also be used with ratio data; in addition, ratio data permits use of additional analyses that the lower level of scales does not.

Analytic Procedures II

Descriptive Statistics

All studies should describe the characteristics of the group being studied. Basic descriptive statistics include frequency distributions, percentages and percentiles, means and standard deviations, and contingency tables (cross-tabulations).

Differences Within the Data

Most often, when you are studying interventions, you want to know whether the differences between groups or observations can be attributed to the intervention or whether they could have occurred by chance alone. For example, if 24 percent of an experimental group of 1,000 men use condoms, compared with only 21 percent of the control group, is this difference **statistically significant** (meaning that you can confidently attribute it to your intervention) or could it have occurred by chance? To answer this question, the researcher performs a statistical test. The three common significance tests that we will discuss are the chi-square (χ^2) test, t test, and analysis of variance (ANOVA, or F test).

All statistical tests of significance assume that differences are produced by chance alone. This assumption is called the **null hypothesis**. The statistical tests tell us the probability that the observed differences could have occurred by chance. This number is called the **significance level**. The convention for writing the significance level is p < followed by the probability that the result could have occurred by chance. Thus, p < .05 means that the probability that the result is due to chance alone is less than 1 in 20. By convention, researchers do not usually reject the null hypothesis unless they find p < .05. Obviously, if you choose a very small p value for your significance level, you decrease the probability of rejecting the null hypothesis.

The statistical test also tells you how often you will be wrong in rejecting the null hypothesis. If p < .05, you will be wrong 5 percent of the time. If p < .75, you will be wrong three-fourths of the time. You will be committing a **Type I error** when the results of the test lead you to reject the null hypothesis when in fact the result was due to chance. You commit a **Type II error** when you accept the null hypothesis when in fact the intervention did affect the results. A small significance level decreases the probability of making a **Type I error**, but increases the probability of making a **Type II error**. A common way to decrease the probability of making a **Type II error** is to hold the significance level constant and increase your sample size (see chapter 8). Variance control techniques such as matching (discussed in chapter 7) should also be used in experimental designs whenever possible.

A common misconception is that statistically significant also means important. This is not true. The difference in condom use of 3 percent in the example above may be statistically significant at the p < .05 level, but an HIV/AIDS program manager might not consider the 3 percentage point improvement in condom use to be important enough to justify the money and effort required to make the necessary change in the program. Similarly, a statistically significant 3 percent point difference in condom use may or may not result in a measurable change in HIV infection. Thus, although the difference may be **statistically** significant, it may not be **programmatically** significant.

When assessing the impact of experimental interventions on program outcomes, a conservative approach for a program manager is to first test for statistical significance. If the study fails to reject the null hypothesis, the manager does not need to make a judgment about the practical importance of the observed difference. However, if the statistical test leads to rejection of the null hypothesis, the manager must take the next step and attempt to make a judgment about the programmatic importance of the statistically significant result.

CHI-SQUARE (χ^2) TEST

The chi-square (χ^2) test is the only significance test that can be used with nominal data. It is also frequently used with ordinal data and can be used with ratio data, but it is less powerful than statistics that make use of the mean and variance of the data.

The chi-square test is used to determine whether frequency distributions differ significantly. When using χ^2 you first prepare a cross-tabulation of the variables. The chi-square test can then be applied to the cross-tabulation to determine whether there is a significant difference between distributions.

For example, in evaluating the efficiency of mass media recruitment for VCT, you might want to learn whether persons self-referred for VCT after hearing a mass media message were more or less likely to be HIV-positive than persons recruited by the program's peer educators. In this case, the null hypothesis to be tested is that there is no difference in HIV status because of the referral source. The chi-square test works by comparing the actually **observed** outcomes to outcomes that would be **expected** if there were no difference between the two groups. The cross-tabulation for this comparison might look as follows:

TABLE 11.1 HIV status differences between clients referred by mass media and clients referred by peer educators for testing

REFERRAL SOURCE	HIV STATUS		
	Positive	Negative	Total
Mass media	25 (4.16%)	575 (95.84%)	600
Peer educator	75 (18.75%)	325 (81.25%)	400
Total	100	900	1000

Only about 4 percent of clients referred by the mass media are HIV-positive. In comparison, almost 19 percent of clients referred by peer educators are HIV-positive. Thus, there is a difference between your groups. They have different rates of seropositivity, but is the difference statistically significant? Since seropositive status is a dichotomous nominal variable, the appropriate test is the χ^2. Similarly, when studying ordinal variables, you might use a chi-square test if you want to learn whether persons with a secondary school or higher education were more likely to "strongly approve" of mass media condom advertising than people with less education.

t TEST OF MEANS

The *t* test is used to determine whether the difference between two means is statistically significant. A *t* test can be used only with interval or ratio data. For example, in an intervention study you would use the *t* test to determine whether intervention clinics saw more clients than control clinics, or whether individuals who attended a two-hour course on HIV/AIDS reduced the number of their sexual partners, compared to persons who did not attend the course.

F TEST (ANALYSIS OF VARIANCE—ANOVA TEST)

The *F* test, or analysis of variance (ANOVA) is usually used to determine whether the difference between three or more means is significant. You would use an ANOVA test whenever you did a multiple group experiment. For example, will peer educators perform better if they are given one, two, or three days of retraining? Both *t* tests and *F* tests require interval or ratio data because they use variance estimates in calculating statistical significance.

Correlations Between Variables

In a descriptive study (a design that does not include an experimental treatment), researchers often look for "correlations" between variables to determine whether there is an underlying relationship between them, or whether one factor (for example, age at positive HIV test) is related to another (such as years of survival) factor. If you have interval or ratio data, you can use **Pearson's correlation coefficient** to measure the degree of association between the variables. When you have ordinal data, **Spearman's** and **Kendall's rank correlation tests** are appropriate for measuring association.

The tests produce numbers called **correlation coefficients** that range from -1.0 to +1.0. When the correlation coefficient is negative (that is, preceded by a minus sign), it means that the relationship is such that one variable decreases as the other increases. In the example above, a negative correlation would mean that the older people are at age of HIV diagnosis, the shorter their survival time, and vice versa. If the correlation coefficient is positive (preceded by a + sign), it means that when one variable is high, so is the other, and that when one variable is low, so is the other.

The closer the correlation coefficient is to +1.0 (or to -1.0), the stronger the relationship or association between the two variables (for example, a correlation of 0.2 implies a weaker relationship than a correlation of 0.7). A correlation coefficient of 0 means that no relationship between the two variables exists, and a coefficient of 1.0 means that the two variables are perfectly related or correlated.

Tests of significance can be applied to the correlation coefficient. However, instead of testing the probability that differences between groups could have been the result of chance, as is the case in making comparisons between experimental groups, measures of association test the probability that the degree of the observed relationship is different from 0.

Be careful to note that correlation does not mean causality. In using correlational techniques, the researcher needs to keep in mind that the correlation between two or more variables does not necessarily imply that variation in one variable causes variation in the other variables. In other words, just because variable A is correlated, associated, or related with variable B does not necessarily mean that variable A causes variable B. To use a silly example, drinking tea is usually associated with the use of sugar and milk. But tea drinking does not cause sugar and milk use; rather, it is only associated with it.

To use an HIV/AIDS example, a statistically reliable positive correlation between reading pamphlets about HIV/AIDS and visiting a VCT center does not permit you to say that reading the pamphlet causes a person to seek VCT. In fact, there are three logically possible relationships between HIV/AIDS counseling and testing and pamphlet reading: (1) HIV/AIDS pamphlet reading may lead to visiting a VCT center, (2) visiting a VCT center may lead to HIV/AIDS pamphlet reading, or (3) the association between visiting a VCT center and pamphlet reading may be caused by a third factor, such as engaging in risky sexual behaviors that may lead to both visiting a VCT center and pamphlet reading. These relationships are diagrammed in Figure 11.3.

FIGURE 11.3 Three possible relationships between pamphlet reading and visiting a VCT center

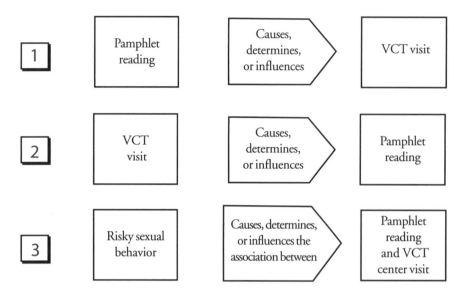

Table 11.2 summarizes the characteristics of the four scales of measurement, and lists appropriate measures of central tendency, variation, comparison, and association for each scale.

TABLE 11.2 Scales of measurement

MEASUREMENT SCALE	EXAMPLES	APPROPRIATE MEASURES OF CENTRAL TENDENCY AND VARIATION	SOME APPROPRIATE MEASURES OF COMPARISON AND ASSOCIATION
NOMINAL	Assigning classes like "HIV-negative" or "HIV-positive" to numbers	Number of cases Mode	Chi-square
ORDINAL	Strength of opinions or beliefs	Median Percentiles Mode Number of cases	Chi-square Tests of rank order correlation
INTERVAL	Fahrenheit and Centigrade scales	Mean Standard deviation Median Percentiles Mode Number of cases	t test Analysis of variance Pearson's r
RATIO	Money, incidence, prevalence, number of visits to a health center, weight, height, knowledge scales	Geometric mean Coefficient of variation Mean Standard deviation Median Percentiles Mode Number of cases	t test Analysis of variance Pearson's r

Multivariate Analysis

Unlike the **bivariate** (only two variables) statistical measurements described above, **multivariate analysis** is used to examine the relationship between more than two variables. Typically, in HIV/AIDS operations research we are concerned with the relationships between multiple independent variables and a single dependent variable. But this is not always the case. Multivariate techniques also exist for examining the relationship between multiple dependent variables and a single independent variable, as well as multiple independent and multiple dependent variables.

In OR, multivariate analysis is sometimes used with quasi-experiments and is often used in descriptive, diagnostic studies. For example, suppose you complete a quasi-experiment to determine whether a training intervention to improve provider competence results in better patient adherence to antiretroviral drug treatment regimens. You perform a *t* test and discover that the patients of providers in the training intervention group have significantly better adherence than did the comparison group. In selecting the intervention and comparison groups, you matched the clinics on the type of antiretroviral treatment regime most often used by patients. However, you did not match the clinics on patient age or education.

When you analyze the data, you find that age and education differences between groups are statistically significant. Our provider training intervention is confounded with patient age and education, which means that the difference in groups may be due to the age or education differences rather than to the training intervention. In this situation, you might be able to separate the effects of client age, education, and provider training by doing a multivariate analysis.

If the relationship between the intervention and adherence continues to be undiminished (statistically significant), even when the other two factors are held constant, you could conclude that age and education have little or no influence on adherence, and you may attribute the differences between groups to provider training. However, if the relationship between provider training and adherence disappears (is no longer statistically significant) when you control for the other two variables, you must conclude that your intervention was not successful in improving patient compliance. In addition to determining which independent variables are significantly related to a dependent variable, multivariate techniques, like simple correlations, may also allow you to measure the strength of the relationship.

In a diagnostic OR study, in contrast to an intervention study, you typically want to know what factors are related to a problem or a behavior. For example, if your problem is relatively poor patient adherence to antiretroviral treatment, you may want to examine the association between adherence and several patient variables, such as gender, age, education, income, and ARV side effects, as well as some clinic variables, such as the complexity of the regimen and frequency of clinic appointments.

There are several multivariate techniques. The one you should use depends, just as with bivariate techniques, on the measurement scale of the variables. The matrix in Table 11.3 shows five of the more commonly used multivariate procedures for different combinations of independent and dependent variables.

TABLE 11.3 Multivariate procedures

MEAUREMENT SCALE OF INDEPENDENT VARIABLES	MEASUREMENT SCALE OF DEPENDENT VARIABLES			
	Dichotomous (two categories)	Nominal (more than two categories)	Ordinal (more than two categories)	Interval and Ratio
Dichotomous, nominal, and ordinal	Logistic regression	Multinomial logistic regression	Multinomial logistic regression ordered	Multiple regression with dummy independent variables
Interval and ratio	Logistic regression	Multinomial logistic regression	Multinomial logistic regression ordered	Multiple regression
Mixed (any combination of measurement scales)	Logistic regression	Multinomial logistic regression	Multinomial logistic regression ordered	Multiple regression

When using multivariate techniques, we often use the term **dummy variables.** A dummy variable, also called a binary variable, is a dichotomous variable for which the two categories are coded as 1 and 0. This coding changes the meaning of the categories. Instead of 1 = hospital and 2 = clinic, the meaning of the dummy variable is 1 = hospital and 0 = not hospital. **Dummy variables** are frequently used in multivariate analysis because they allow researchers to treat nominal and ordinal variables as interval variables in using statistical tests.

NOMINAL DEPENDENT VARIABLE

Suppose you are trying to learn the determinants of where people go for VCT. The dependent variable, "Site where VCT received," could be treated as a nominal measurement by asking the question "Where did you go for your VCT?" and offering the following response categories: 1 = hospital, 2 = urban clinic, 3 = rural health center.

With a nominal dependent variable with three or more categories, you can use a technique called "**multinomial logistic regression.**" As in logistic regression, the variable is transformed into a type of measure called a "binary logit," which can be thought of as being similar to a dummy variable. Then the multinomial technique regresses each independent variable on all the possible outcome comparisons: 1 versus 2, 2 versus 3, and 1 versus 3.

The multinomial regression then tells us how the independent variable, say, place of residence, affects the **odds**, or **probability**, that a person will choose 1 over 2, 2 over 3, or 1 over 3.

ORDINAL DEPENDENT VARIABLE

Returning to our example of adherence as a dependent variable, you could measure adherence on an ordinal scale with the following question, "During the last month how frequently did you miss taking your medication?" with these response categories: 1 = not at all frequently, 2 = somewhat frequently, and 3 = very frequently. You could use the multinomial regression technique used with nominal independent variables or the more efficient **ordered logistic regression** model.

In the typical operations research application, you would use the ordered model to determine how an independent variable affects the probability of a given response (for example, how age affects the probability of responding "not at all frequently"). You can use this technique to estimate how much a one-unit change in the independent variable affects the probability of a response while holding all other independent variables constant. You might find that a one-year increase in age increases the probability of not taking the medication "not at all frequently" by .03.

INTERVAL/RATIO DEPENDENT VARIABLE

Whenever the dependent variable is interval or ratio, the **multiple regression** technique can be used, regardless of the measurement scales of the independent variables. Perhaps the most common type of multivariate analysis used in HIV/AIDS research is multiple regression with a ratio level dependent variable and a combination of ratio and dummy coded nominal variables.

CAUTION !

Multivariate techniques can be very powerful analytical tools, but they must be used with great care. Always keep in mind that experiments rather than multivariate analyses are the preferred method for demonstrating that an intervention (the independent variable) **causes** a difference in the dependent variable. Multivariate analyses, at best, only approximate the control afforded by a true experimental design.

Consequently, multivariate analyses should be used to study causality only when random assignment is impossible. For example, if you want to demonstrate that injecting drug use causes HIV infection, you would have to rely on a multivariate analysis because you cannot ethically assign individuals to inject drugs.

Moreover, multivariate techniques, even when used with descriptive studies, are all based on numerous assumptions, at least some of which are usually not met. As a result, apparent findings often are not valid. Multivariate statistics can also be difficult to understand for many managers without a research background. Your plan of analysis should avoid multivariate techniques unless you are already well acquainted with them or can call on the assistance of an experienced consultant who can both perform the statistical test *and* accurately interpret the results from the test.

Cost-effectiveness Analysis

All HIV/AIDS programs cost money, which pays for program activities, which are designed to produce desired results or outcomes. Because resources are limited, programs must make decisions about the most effective way to spend available funds. To help managers make decisions about the affordability of a proposed intervention, operations research projects often include **cost-effectiveness analysis (CEA)**, which allows the decision maker to choose between two or more alternatives on the basis of both the costs and results of each alternative.

The cost-effectiveness of an alternative is the ratio of its costs to its outcomes. The result of dividing costs by outcomes produces a measure of the cost per unit of the same outcome (e.g., HIV infections detected) or effectiveness measure.

$$\text{Cost per unit of outcome} = \frac{\text{Costs}}{\text{Outcomes}}$$

The difference in cost per unit of outcome among alternatives can be affected by either a difference in costs, a difference in outcomes, or a difference in both costs and outcomes. Ideally outcomes in CEA should be indicators of population or individual level health status, such as HIV incidence or prevalence, or years of survival after diagnosis of HIV/AIDS. In practice, however, we usually settle for some intermediate outcome such as number of HIV tests, an increase in knowledge or condom use, or a decrease in the number of sexual partners.

Most often, in an operations research project we are concerned with whether the **additional** costs of a new activity are justified by the number of **additional** outcomes resulting from the activity. For example, suppose the Ministry of Health is considering expanding the existing, health-center-based system of HIV testing to include testing in secondary schools. In deciding if it's worthwhile to add school-based testing, the decision maker would probably want to know how much the expansion would cost, how many additional cases of HIV would be detected among secondary school students, and what the cost per additional case detected would be. This type of analysis is called an **incremental cost-effectiveness analysis (ICEA)**. The incremental cost effectiveness ratio is calculated as:

$$\frac{\text{Incremental cost}}{\text{per unit of outcome}} = \frac{\text{Additional costs}}{\text{Additional outcomes}}$$

The costs used in the **incremental cost effectiveness ratio (ICER)** are only the costs associated with adding services to secondary schools, and the outcomes are only the number of positives detected in the secondary school testing sites.

PLAN THE CEA WHEN YOU FIRST DESIGN THE STUDY

Like any other analysis, **you must begin planning for a CEA at the time you design your study.** Do not try to design your CEA after the rest of the study is complete. You will not be able to obtain all the data needed in the time needed, and the analysis is liable to give misleading results.

After deciding on what the study outcome is, you must identify the costs that go into producing that outcome. You must also identify **where** and **how** you will obtain the cost data, who will collect it, and what computer program (usually a spreadsheet) will be used to process the cost data and calculate the cost-effectiveness ratios.

When preparing an OR proposal that includes CEA be sure to mention the following:

- Is the analysis comparing total costs and outcomes or only incremental costs and outcomes?
- What types of data will be collected?
- When will the data be collected, by whom, and with what data collection instruments?

Before doing a cost-effectiveness analysis, read a manual or a text devoted to this topic. Aside from the general citations in the bibliography, the researcher may wish to consult the 1998 technical update from UNAIDS, *Costing Guidelines for HIV Prevention* (see references).

To obtain data on costs, we usually look at the following five general program cost categories:
- Labor (salaries and benefits).
- Materials and supplies.
- Capital items (vehicles, computers, printers, and furniture).
- Infrastructure (buildings, rent, and utilities).
- Indirect costs or overhead.

These costs must be obtained from actual program records or observations and not from budgets. The number of inputs and their actual cost will probably be different from what is estimated in a program budget. The actual calculations of costs are usually simple. However, the identification of costs and the decisions that must be made about them can be quite complex.

The cost analyst must ensure that all relevant program costs are taken into account. Program personnel may include the time of janitors, service providers, and others. Materials and supplies include both medical supplies and office supplies. In gathering data, the cost analyst may also have to make decisions about the cost of items that are used by many different facilities or programs. For example, if a laboratory technician performs many tests other than those used to diagnose HIV infection, you will have to decide how to apportion the time and cost associated with doing HIV tests from the time and costs associated with other, non-HIV-related tests. This and many other decisions are crucial in doing any type of CEA.

In HIV/AIDS operations research, CEA is usually done as part of the analysis of an experiment or quasi-experiment that compares a new program intervention to a traditional intervention. In this situation, we must be sure to calculate the following sets of costs:

The cost of designing the intervention, including labor, materials, consultants, overhead, and any other relevant items. These costs may be related to meetings and time spent designing new materials.

The cost of implementing the intervention, including any training and supervision costs, and any additional personnel, supply, or capital costs. If the intervention results in attracting additional clients or clinic visits or in performing more tests, then the analyst must include the costs of the additional services provided in the cost of implementing the intervention.

The cost-effectiveness of the intervention in an experimental study. Since the impact of the new intervention will be expected to last beyond the study period, all design and many implementation costs will have to be annualized over the period that the benefits of the intervention are estimated to occur, and not for just the study period. The dependent variable in the study should be used as the effectiveness or outcome measure in the CEA. Finally, the analyst must exclude all research costs from the analysis.

Dummy Tables

Constructing dummy tables is a very useful way to visualize how data can be organized and summarized. A dummy table contains all the elements of a real table, except that the cells of the table are empty (see Table 11.4 for an example). In an OR proposal, the major relationships between variables should be shown in dummy tables.

Cross-tabulation tables are usually presented with cell frequencies converted into percentages based on either row or column totals. If a dependent variable is cross-tabulated with an independent variable, the percentages should be calculated so that they add up to 100 percent for each category of the indepen-

dent variable. For example, in the dummy table presented below, the percentage totals are calculated for the categories of the independent variable ("presence of peer educators in village"). Note also that in tables of this kind, it is always important to present the N, or number of cases that are used to calculate the percentages. You will recall that earlier we noted that it is not a good idea to calculate a percent on an N value that is less than 50.

TABLE 11.4
Example of a dummy table: level of condom use at last intercourse in 100 villages by the presence of peer educators in the village

| LEVEL OF CONDOM USE AT LAST INTERCOURSE | PRESENCE OF PEER EDUCATOR IN VILLAGE | | |
	No (N=)	Yes (N=)	All villages (N=)
50+ percent			
25-49 percent			
0-24 percent			
Total percent	100	100	100

What To Do: The Plan of Analysis

1. Describe in detail each of the analytical techniques and statistical measures you plan to use, indicating how each technique and measure will help you meet your study objectives. What variables will be involved? Why have you selected a particular technique for the analysis of the data?

2. Provide examples of important dummy tables.

3. Be sure that your plan of analysis clearly explains how you will meet all your study objectives, use all your study variables, and test all your study hypotheses.

CHAPTER 12

DISSEMINATION AND UTILIZATION OF RESEARCH FINDINGS

There is very little reason to conduct research unless the results are communicated to others in a form that is both understandable and usable. At the beginning of this *Handbook,* we defined operations research as a **continuous process with five basic steps.** The last two steps are **information dissemination** and **information utilization.** The process of operations research is not complete unless you have given as much attention to these last two steps as you have given to the first three.

Dissemination Strategy

Operations research is conducted primarily to provide useful information to program administrators and policymakers so that improvements needed in service delivery can be made. To ensure that an OR study has the maximum impact, you need to plan a dissemination strategy that answers these three critical questions:

- Who are the potential users of the findings from the operations research study?
- Which particular findings will be of most interest to each potential user group?
- What are the best media channels to reach each potential user group?

Usually, the audience or users of OR study findings will be groups ranging from top policymakers and administrators to academicians, mid-level managers, field workers, and users of services. You will need to match the message (findings) with the audience. Some of the findings will be of more interest to one group than to another. To complicate matters, some channels of communication will be more appropriate for reaching one group than for another. The primary purpose of a **dissemination strategy** is to identify the most effective media channel(s) to reach different audience (user) groups with study findings most relevant to their needs.

Typically, a good strategy will involve multiple media channels used repeatedly over a period of time to reach the largest audience possible. For example, there are many different ways to disseminate information. There is the final study report, which usually will be read by only a limited number of very interested stakeholders. Other ways to disseminate findings include short one- or two-page research summaries, oral presentations at meetings, posters at professional meetings, a stakeholders' end-of-study seminar, internet web page reports, press releases, professional journal articles, and small group meetings with key program managers.

A good dissemination strategy is to have frequent small meetings with key managers and other stakeholders throughout the research process, to keep them informed about study developments. This strategy may reinforce the stakeholders' support for the study and make later use of results more likely. Frequent small meetings will also allow you to anticipate questions and concerns that will be raised at final seminars or about final reports.

Writing Reports

Although research findings can be disseminated in a number of different ways, at a minimum all OR studies should be presented in one or more written reports. The reports should be written in a style that is appropriate for a particular audience.

If the audience is program managers, remember that they are usually not research methodologists. Technical material on sampling, study design, and similar issues should not clutter the report and obscure important findings. Technical material can always be put in an appendix (or several appendices) rather than in the body of the report.

Sometimes managers find it difficult to see the relevance of research findings to program administration and improvement. You should help them by pointing out the implications you think the findings have for program change and improvement. Include in your report recommendations for program change that the data suggest.

One of the major complaints of managers is that research reports are needlessly complex, take too long to come out, and are outdated by the time they appear. Try to avoid this criticism by releasing interim reports as soon as relevant findings become available. Write an **Executive Summary** of the main report. In the Executive Summary, it is not necessary for you to talk about, for example, how the OR study used a quasi-experimental, non-equivalent control group design to obtain data that were analyzed using multivariate analysis. Focus instead on major findings that have implications for program improvement. Use simple, easy-to-understand graphics to present data and simple language that avoids research jargon.

An effective way to disseminate important findings to program managers is to hold an end-of-study seminar. The seminar can be used not only as a forum to disseminate important findings, but also as a means of involving program managers and other stakeholders in a discussion of the meaning of the data and of how the findings can be used to make needed program improvements. The recommendations from the seminar can also be included as an important part of the final operations research study report.

If a report is being written for a more academically oriented group of professionals, the format of the report will be quite different from that used with program managers. The report should be written so that readers can judge the scientific value of the study, assess the adequacy of the study design, and, if they want, repeat the study in other areas or with other subjects.

Example of Major Headings for a Final Research Report

- Title page (title of the report, authors, institutional affiliation, and date of publication).
- Preface (acknowledgments, source of funding).
- Abstract or Executive Summary (which should be short, clear, and concise).
- Background (location of study, special circumstances of study).
- Literature review.
- Study methodology (objectives, hypotheses, description of program intervention, study design, data collection procedures, analytic procedures, limitations of study).
- Findings.
- Discussion of findings and program implications.
- Conclusions and recommendations.
- References and bibliography.
- Appendices.

What To Do: Reporting Research Findings

Include a section in your research proposal that describes your plan for disseminating information. The plan should specify the following:

1. Who the potential users of the findings are.

2. Which particular findings will be of most interest to each user group.

3. Which media channels will be used to reach each group.

Utilization of Study Findings

The utilization of research results is the goal of every OR activity. Unfortunately, it is often a goal that is not fully realized. One reason is that the people who design and implement operations research studies are usually not the same people who use the results. A second reason is that sometimes the researchers mistakenly believe that a study is completed when the final report is written and disseminated. As noted earlier, the process of operations research is not complete until the results are disseminated fully and every effort has been made to have them used. A basic and very important part of the OR process is to see that the results from OR studies are used.

Utilization simply means making use of something. For operations research, the "something" is either study results or the study process. There are many ways that the study results or process can be used. For example, senior government officials can use OR findings to formulate or redirect policies on national health and HIV/AIDS. Directors of service delivery agencies can use OR findings for strategic planning. NGOs and community-based organizations can use OR findings to improve services that are provided to PLHA or others affected by HIV/AIDS such as orphans.

The process of conducting an operations research study can also be used to identify key problem areas in programs and focus attention and resources on solving these problems. Similarly, researchers can use OR findings to refine social science theory, and they can use the process of study implementation to develop new data collection or analysis techniques and to train young researchers. Field supervisors and field workers as well as clinic personnel can use OR findings to evaluate their own performance and improve the quality of service delivery. The findings from intervention

OR studies can be used to expand and scale up program activities for a larger geographic area or to reach more people.

It is unusual to find situations in which OR study results are accepted wholly and completely and implemented immediately to change an entire service delivery system. Rather, OR study results are combined with other information (such as political and experiential information, a colleague's opinion, or other research findings) to provide a more complete picture of a situation. The new information could be crucial, particularly if it provides decision makers with the additional confidence they need to make necessary service delivery changes. In some cases, "utilization" does not refer to the use of results from studies, but instead to the use of an operations research process that identifies and defines problems and systematically examines potential strategies for overcoming these problems.

Although there is no way researchers can guarantee that study results will be used by decision makers, they can do a number of things to greatly increase the probability of utilization. Examples of these are listed below:

- When a study is being planned, identify a very specific list of decision makers most likely to be interested in the study topic. Contact these people and fully inform them about the objectives of the study. They are the stakeholders who need to feel "ownership" of the study. They should be actively involved in helping to formulate the objectives of the study, assisting with the implementation, and interpreting the results from the study.

- Develop a plan for involving the potential users of the results in all aspects of the study. The more actively involved they are in the planning, implementation, and analysis of a study, the more likely they will be to commit to using the study's results. Identify specific times when the key stakeholders can meet to review the progress of the study and participate in the major decisions related to it.

- Interim and final study reports should include a section on "Study Implications." Indicate clearly and succinctly what you and the major stakeholders believe are the action implications that are likely to arise from the study.

- At end-of-study seminars, provide sufficient time for participants to discuss fully the results from the study and to develop an action plan for using the results. This can sometimes be done by dividing the participants into small groups.

What To Do: Utilization of Study Results

In your study proposal, include a section on the utilization of the study's findings. In this section you should:

1. Identify the organizations you believe will be most interested in the study.

2. Discuss how you will involve these organizations in the various planning, implementation, analysis, and dissemination stages of the study.

3. Indicate what you believe will be the policy or program implications most likely to arise from the study.

CHAPTER 13

LIMITATIONS OF THE STUDY

One of the most important responsibilities of researchers is to report on the limitations and problems in their study. When you know of problems and limitations before you are starting a study, you should discuss them in the operations research proposal. (You should report these and any additional problems that occur during the research in the write-up of the study.) **Never try to conceal or misrepresent limitations and problems.**

Design and Analysis Limitations

There is no such thing as a perfect study. Every research study has some problems with the reliability and validity of the data, the size of the sample, the questionnaire design, the implementation, or the analysis plan. Good research attempts to keep these problems to a minimum, but some problems will always remain.

Remember that the researcher can commit sins of both commission and omission. In a research study proposal, it is best to recognize the limitations of your design rather than try to pretend that these limitations do not exist. For example, if you have purposively selected a study sample, do not try to pretend that this sample is representative of a much larger group. If you are forced, because of limited time and funds, to use data that may be of questionable quality (such as clinic records or service statistics), do not try to pretend that the data are completely reliable and valid. If your comparison and control groups are not equivalent, do not try to pretend that they are. Point out to the reader the problems in your study design and discuss the reasons that you think the study should be conducted despite the inevitable problems.

Special Situational Factors

In your proposal, mention any special situations that might influence the study. In Asia and other areas of the world, for example, it is often difficult to conduct field studies during the rainy season. If this is a problem, say that the study can be conducted only in months when heavy rain does not occur. If doing your study depends on prior approval from senior government officials (which often can cause long delays), mention this fact in the proposal.

What To Do: Limitations of the Study

Be frank about the limitations of your study and the possible situational factors that might influence the results of the study. Mention these limitations both in the proposal and in the final report.

CHAPTER 14

RESOURCES AND FACILITIES

Available Resources and Facilities Available

Most reviewers of study proposals will want to know what resources and facilities will be available for conducting the research. For example, are experienced interviewers and coders available? Is appropriate software available? Will other institutions or organizations contribute to the funding of the study? What are the qualifications of the principal investigator and how much of his or her time will be devoted to the study—for example, 100 percent, 50 percent, or 10 percent? These and similar questions about the availability of resources and facilities should be addressed in the proposal. It is customary for the budget to be included in the final section of a proposal before the appendices.

Study Budget

The budget for the research study should be realistic and should be confined to those items really necessary to conduct the study. In general, most research donors will not provide money for expensive equipment, building construction, or vehicles. Moreover, donors probably will not provide salary payments to research staff that are above what they have received on other jobs. Any local contributions or large and unusual items in the budget should be explained and justified. Be very clear about each cost item in the budget. Show the components of the item. For example, if you plan to employ interviewers, you might show their salary costs as follows:

Interviewers (20 persons at   Rs 200,000
Rs 500 per day x 20 days)

Arrange the budget under major cost categories (see Figure 14.1). If your study extends beyond a year, show first-year costs separately from second-year costs. Finally, if the research is to be supported by international donor funding, you may be required to itemize costs in both local currency and the currency of the donor.

What To Do: Resources and Facilities

1. Describe the resources and facilities available for the study. Be sure to indicate:

   • Whether other institutions or organizations will contribute resources.
   • The availability of computers, trained interviewers and coders, secretarial help, vehicles, office space, and so on that will be needed to implement the research.

2. For the study budget, arrange the cost items under headings. Major headings should include the following:

   • Salaries and benefits.
   • Materials, supplies, and equipment.
   • Travel and per-diem.
   • Report publication and dissemination.

3. At the end of the budget, explain and justify any large or unusual cost items.

FIGURE 14.1
Example of a study budget to be submitted to an
international donor for a project in Thailand

ITEMIZED RESEARCH BUDGET

	Thai baht (B)	US dollars ($)
A. Salaries and benefits		
1. Principal investigator, 1 (50% time), B15,000/mo. x 12 mos.	180,000	4,091
2. Associate investigator, 1 (100% time) B20,000/mo. x 12 mos.	240,000	5,455
3. Field interviewers, 20 @B600/day x 10 days	120,000	2,727
4. Secretarial services, 1 (25% time) B8,000/mo. x 12 mos.	96,000	2,182
Subtotal	636,000	14,454
B. Travel and per-diem		
1. Air-fare, 6 round trips Bangkok-Chiang Mai @ B5000 ea.	30,000	682
2. Local transportation (bus), Chiang Mai 20 interviewers @B100/day x 10 days	20,000	455
3. Per-diem (investigators), Chiang Mai B400 x 18 person days	7,200	164
Subtotal	57,200	1,300
C. Materials and Supplies		
1. Questionnaire printing, 1,000 @ B15 ea.	15,000	341
2. Pencils, computer paper, diskettes	4,000	91
3. Printing of final report 200 copies @B100 ea.	20,000	455
Subtotal	39,000	886
D. Dissemination seminar	12,000	273
Total Cost	744,200	16,914

Exchange rate: Baht 44 = US$1.00 (11/10/01)

An Example of a Budget Justification

LOCAL CONTRIBUTIONS

The Thailand Ministry of Health will provide office space, equipment (including computers and software), communications, and utilities for the duration of the project. Study data will be entered into the computer and cleaned by Ministry data entry staff at no cost to the project.

SALARIES AND BENEFITS

The principal investigator is a full-time member of the operations research faculty of The Royal University. She will be employed half-time by the project at her regular university salary level rate. The money will be paid directly to the university to cover the costs of replacement faculty who will assume her teaching duties for one year. The principal investigator's salary will also continue to be paid by the university. Similarly, the secretary is an employee of the operations research department of the university. She will be released to work on this study under the same conditions as the principal investigator (see Resources and Facilities Manual, which includes the relevant personnel policies of The Royal University and a copy of the principal investigator's and the secretary's 2000 tax returns, attesting to their salary levels). The associate investigator has recently earned his doctorate in public health from Mahidol University. This is his first job and he will be paid at the rate of a new faculty member at The Royal University (see Resources and Facilities Manual, which contains the Mahidol faculty salary schedule). Field interviewers will be paid at the daily rate authorized by the Ministry of Health.

TRAVEL AND PER-DIEM

The principal investigator will spend three days in Chiang Mai preparing field work with local health authorities. She will also visit Chiang Mai for one day to attend the final project seminar. The associate researcher will spend 14 days in Chiang Mai.

Thirteen of these days will be used to supervise field interviewing and field editing and one day will be used to attend the final seminar. Per-diem rates are those authorized by the Ministry of Health for Chiang Mai.

MATERIALS AND SUPPLIES

Costs of printing are based on three independent bids.

DISSEMINATION SEMINAR

The costs of the final seminar include rental of a meeting room at the Chiang Mai Imperial Hotel and a tea break for 100 persons.

CHAPTER 15

APPENDICES

Include in the appendices of your proposal any additional information you think might be helpful to a proposal reviewer. For example, include:

- Biographical data on the principal investigators.

- The study questionnaire if you have it.

- The Informed Consent Form.

- A copy of the approval from the Institutional Review Board.

- Any explanatory material (such as an annual report) about your institution or the organization under whose name the study will be conducted.

- A list of references in the appendices, if you have cited literature in the proposal.

CHAPTER 16

TITLE PAGE AND ABSTRACT

Although the title page and abstract appear as the first section of a research proposal, they are the last to be written. The title page (see example below) gives the essential information about the proposal. Immediately following the title page you should include an abstract. The abstract is a summary of the basic information contained in all the other sections of your proposal.

Do not overload an abstract with unnecessary information. Keep it short (no longer than one or two pages), precise, and to the point. The abstract should tell the reader:

- **The problem** to be studied.

- The main **objectives** of the study.

- The major expected **implications** of the study.

- **Who** will conduct the study.

- **When** the study will be conducted.

- **Where** the study will be conducted.

- **What methods** will be used to conduct the study.

- **What resources** are required for the study.

What To Do: Title Page and Abstract

1. Write one or two sentences that give the essence of the information in each major section of your completed proposal.

2. Arrange the sentences into an abstract so that the text is clear and easy to understand.

3. Attach a title page to the abstract.

Example of a Title Page

HIV/AIDS Operations Research Proposal

Title: An Experimental Operations Research Study to Promote Dual Protection by Integrating HIV/AIDS Activities with a Family Planning Program

Location: **Kisumu, Kenya**

Sponsoring institution(s):   **The Institute for Rural, Social, and Health Development (IRSHD)**

Principal investigator(s):   **Dr. George Ndeti**
                                    Director
                                    IRSHD
                                    Nairobi, Kenya

Starting date: **April 2002**

Completion date: **June 2005**

Total cost: US$65,471

BIBLIOGRAPHY

Academy for Educational Development (AED). 1998. *Critical Issues in HIV Prevention Evaluation: A Monograph*. Washington, DC: AED.

AIDS Control and Prevention Project. 1997. *Making Prevention Work: Global Lessons Learned from the AIDS Control and Prevention (AIDSCAP) Project, 1991–1997*. Arlington, VA: Family Health International.

Andrews, Frank M. et al. *A Guide for Selecting Statistical Techniques for Analyzing Social Science Data*. Ann Arbor, MI: Institute for Social Research.

Andrews, Frank M. et al. 1975. *Multiple Classification Analysis* (2nd ed.). Ann Arbor, MI: Institute for Social Research.

Babbie, Earl R. 1979. "Content analysis and the analysis of existing data," in *The Practice of Social Research*. Belmont, CA: Wadsworth, pp. 232–264.

Berelson, Bernard. 1971. *Content Analysis in Communication Research*. New York: Hafner.

Bertrand, Jane T., J. Stover, and R. Porter. 1989. "Methodologies for evaluating the impact of contraceptive social marketing programs." *Evaluation Review* 13.

Bickman, Leonard and Debra J. Rog (eds.). 1998. *Handbook of Applied Social Research Methods*. Thousand Oaks, CA: Sage.

Blalock, Hubert M., Jr. 1970. *An Introduction to Social Research*. Englewood Cliffs, NJ: Prentice-Hall General Sociology Series.

———. 1971. *Causal Models in the Social Sciences*. Chicago: Aldine-Atherton.

———. 1972. *Social Statistics* (2nd ed.). New York: McGraw-Hill.

Blalock, Hubert M., Jr. and Ann B. Blalock. 1968. *Methodology in Social Research*. New York: McGraw-Hill.

Blumenfeld, Stewart N. 1985. *Operations Research Methods: A General Approach to Primary Health Care*. Chevy Chase, MD: PRICOR.

Boerma, J. Ties et al. 2001. "Measurement of biomarkers in surveys in developing countries: Opportunities and problems." *Population and Development Review* 27(2): 303–314.

Box, George E. P. et al. 1978. *Statistics for Experimenters*. New York: John Wiley and Sons.

Brown, Steven R. and Lawrence E. Melamed. 1990. *Experimental Design and Analysis*. Thousand Oaks, CA: Sage.

Campbell, Donald T. and Julian C. Stanley. 1963. *Experimental and Quasi-Experimental Designs for Research*. Chicago: Rand McNally.

Caraël, M. 1995. "Sexual behavior," in *Sexual Behavior and AIDS in the Developing World*. J. Cleland and B. Ferry, eds. London: Taylor & Francis.

Catania, J. 1990a. "Response bias in assessing sexual behaviors relevant to HIV transmission." *Evaluation Program Planner* 13.

———. 1990b. "Methodological problems in AIDS behavioral research: Influences on measurement error and participation bias in studies of sexual behavior." *Psychology Bulletin* 3.

Centers for Disease Control and Prevention (CDC). 1998. *HIV Prevention Evaluation Guidance*. Atlanta: CDC.

Coates, R.A. et al. 1986. "The reliability of sexual histories in AIDS-related research: Evaluation of an interview –administered questionnaire." *Canadian Journal of Public Health* 77(5).

Coates, Thomas et al. 1988. "Behavioral factors in the spread of HIV Infection." *AIDS* 2 (Supplement 1): S239–246.

Coates, Thomas et al. 1996. "HIV prevention in developed countries." *Lancet* 348: 1143–48.

Coates, Thomas et al. 2000. "Efficacy of voluntary HIV-1 counseling and testing individuals and couples in Kenya, Tanzania and Trinidad: A randomized trial." *Lancet* 356(9224): 103.

Cochran, W. G. and G. M. Cox. 1957. *Experimental Designs* (2nd ed.). New York: John Wiley and Sons.

Cohen, Jacob. 1980. *Statistical Power Analysis for the Behavioral Sciences* (2nd ed.). Hillsdale, NJ: Lawrence Erlbaum Associates.

Cook, Thomas D. and Donald T. Campbell. 1979. *Quasi-Experimentation: Design and Analysis Issues for Field Settings*. Chicago: Rand McNally.

Coyle, S., R. Bourch, and C. Turner. 1991. *Evaluating AIDS Prevention Programs*. Washington: National Academy Press.

Creese, A. and D. Parker (eds.). 1994. *Cost Analysis in Primary Health Care: A Training Manual for Programme Managers*. Geneva: WHO.

Demographic and Health Surveys. 1997. *Model B Questionnaire*. Calverton, MD: DHS-III Basic Documentation, Macro International, Inc.

Demographic and Health Surveys. 1997. *Interviewer's Manual for Use with Model "B" Questionnaire*. Calverton, MD: DHS-III Basic Documentation, Macro International, Inc.

Demographic and Health Surveys. 1997. *Supervisor's and Editor's Manual for Use with Model "A" and "B" Questionnaires*. Calverton, MD: DHS-III Basic Documentation, Macro International, Inc.

De Zoysa, I. et al. 1995. "Role of HIV counseling and testing in changing risk behavior in developing countries." *AIDS* 9 (Supplement A): S95–101.

Family Health International. 2002. *Research Ethics Training Curriculum* (CD-ROM). Research Triangle Park, NC: Family Health International.

Fishbein, M. and W. Pequegnat. 2000. "Evaluating AIDS prevention interventions using behavioral and biological outcome measures." *Sexually Transmitted Diseases* 27(2).

Fisher, Andrew A. et al. 1991. *Handbook for Family Planning Operations Research Design: Second Edition.* New York: Population Council.

Fisher, Andrew A., John Laing, and John Stoeckel. 1985. "Guidelines for overcoming design problems in family planning operations research." *Studies in Family Planning* 16(2).

Fisher, Andrew A. and Raymond Carlaw. 1985. "Family planning field research: Balancing internal against external validity." *Studies in Family Planning* 14(1).

Fitz-Gibbon, Carol Taylor, and Lynn Lyons Morris. 1978. *How to Calculate Statistics.* Beverly Hills: Sage.

Foreit, James R. and Tomas Frejka (eds.). 1998. *Family Planning Operations Research: A Book of Readings.* New York: Population Council.

Gilks, C. et al. 1998. *Sexual Health and Health Care: Care and Support for People with HIV/AIDS in Resource Poor Settings.* London: Department of Development.

Gilson, L. et al. 1997. "Cost-effectiveness of improved treatment services for sexually transmitted diseases in preventing HIV-1 infection in Mwanza Region, Tanzania." *Lancet* 350: 1,805–1,809.

Gold, Marthe R. et al. (eds.). 1996. *Cost Effectiveness in Health and Medicine.* New York: Oxford University Press.

Grosskurth, Heiner et al. 2000. "Control of sexually transmitted diseases for HIV-1 Prevention: Understanding the Implications of the Mwanza and Rakai trials." *Lancet* 355: 9, 219.

Grosskurth, Heiner et al. 1995. "Impact of improved treatment of sexually transmitted diseases on HIV infection in rural Tanzania: randomized controlled trial." *Lancet* 346: 530–536.

Haladyna, Thomas M. 1994. *Developing and Validating Multiple-Choice Test Items.* Hillsdale, NJ: Lawrence Earlbaum Associates.

Hanenberg, R.S., W. Rojanapithayakorn, and P. Kunasol. 1994. "Impact of Thailand's HIV-control programme as indicated by the decline in sexually transmitted diseases." *Lancet* 334: 243–245.

Hart, Chris. 1998. *Doing a Literature Review: Releasing the Social Science Research Imagination.* London: Sage.

Hogel, J. and M. Sweat. 1996. "Qualitative methods for evaluation research in HIV/AIDS prevention programming." *AIDSCAP Evaluation Tools, Module 5.* Arlington, VA: Family Health International.

Kaleeba, N. et al. 1997. "Participatory evaluation of counseling, medical and social services of The AIDS Support Organization (TASO) in Uganda." *AIDS Care* 9.

Kalton, G. 1989. *Introduction to Sampling.* Newbury Park, CA: Sage.

———. 1993. *Sampling Rare and Elusive Populations.* New York: United Nations, Department for Economic and Social Information and Policy Analysis.

Kerlinger, Fred N. 1964. *Foundations of Behavioral Research.* New York: Holt, Rinehart and Winston.

Kilmarx, Peter H. et al. 2001. "Protection of human subjects' rights in HIV-preventive clinical trials in Africa and Asia: Experiences and recommendations." *AIDS* 15 (Supplement 5): S73–79.

Kirkwood, Betty R. et al. 1997. "Issues in the design and interpretation of studies to evaluate the impact of community-based interventions." *Tropical Medicine and International Health* 11(2): 1,022-1,029.

Kish, Leslie. 1965. *Survey Sampling*. New York: John Wiley and Sons.

Konings, E.G. et al. 1995. "Validating population surveys for the measurement of HIV/STD prevention indicators." *AIDS* 9(4).

Lamptey, Peter, Paul Zeitz, and Carol Larivee (eds.). 2001. *Strategies for an Expanded and Comprehensive Response to a National HIV/AIDS Epidemic: A Handbook for Designing and Implementing HIV/AIDS Programs*. Arlington, VA: Family Health International.

Levin, Henry M. 1983. *Cost-Effectiveness: A Primer*. Thousand Oaks, CA: Sage.

Lewis-Beck, Michael S. 1980. *Applied Regression: An Introduction*. Beverly Hills: Sage Publications.

Lilienfeld, Abraham and David E. Lilenfeld. 1980. *Foundations of Epidemiology*. New York: Oxford University Press.

Loue, Sana. 2000. *Textbook of Research Ethics, Theory and Practice*. New York: Klewer Academic/Plenum Publishers.

Mann, J., L. et al. 1994. "Health and human rights." *Health and Human Rights* 1(1).

McDowell, Ian and Claire Newell. 1996. *Measuring Health: A Guide to Rating Scales and Questionnaires*. New York: Oxford University Press.

Mertens, T.E. and M. Caraël. 1997. "Evaluation of HIV/STD prevention, care and support: An update on WHO's approaches." *AIDS Education Preview* 9(2).

Miller, Kate et al. 1998. *Clinic-Based Family Planning and Reproductive Health Services in Africa: Findings from Situation Analysis Studies*. New York: Population Council.

Miller, Robert, Andy Fisher et al. 1997. *The Situation Analysis Approach to Assessing Family Planning and Reproductive Health Services: A Handbook*. New York: Population Council.

Mills, S. et al. 1998. "HIV risk behavioral surveillance: A methodology for monitoring behavioral trends." *AIDS* 12 (Supplement 2).

Oakley, Ann. 1998. "Experimentation and social interventions: A forgotten but important history." *British Medical Journal* 317: 1,239-1,242.

Patton, Michael Quinn. 1978. *Utilization-Focused Evaluation*. Beverly Hills, CA: Sage.

———. 1980. *Qualitative Evaluation Methods*. Beverly Hills, CA: Sage.

———. 1990. *Qualitative Evaluation and Research Methods* (2nd ed.). Newbury Park, CA: Sage.

Rehle, Thomas. et al. 1998. "AVERT: A user-friendly model to estimate the impact of HIV/sexually transmitted disease prevention interventions on HIV transmission." *AIDS* 12 (Supplement 2).

Rehle, Thomas et al. 2001. *Evaluating Programs for HIV/AIDS Prevention and Care in Developing Countries: A Handbook for Program Managers and Decision Makers*. Arlington, VA: Family Health International.

Reynolds, Richard and K. Celeste Gaspari. 1985. "Cost-effectiveness analysis," *PRICOR Monograph Series, Methods Paper No. 2.* Chevy Chase, MD: Center for Human Services.

Ringheim, Karin. 1995. "Ethical issues in social science research with special reference to sexual behavior research." *Social Science and Medicine* 40(12): 1,691–1,697.

Rossi, Peter H. and and Howard E. Freeman. 1982. *Evaluation: A Systematic Approach*. Beverly Hills, CA: Sage.

Rossi, Peter H. and Howard E. Freeman. 1990. *Evaluation: A Systematic Approach* (5th ed.). Newbury Park, CA: Sage.

Saidel, T. et al. 1998. "Indicators and the measurement of STD case management in developing countries." *AIDS* 12 (Supplement 2).

Selltiz, Claire et al. 1959. *Research Methods in Social.* New York: Holt, Rinehart and Winston.

Sewankambo, Nelson K. et al. 1994. "Demographic impact of HIV infection in rural Rakai District, Uganda: Results of a population-based cohort study." *AIDS* 8: 1,707–1,713.

Siegel, Sidney. 1956. *Nonparametric Statistics for the Behavioral Sciences*. New York: McGraw-Hill.

Snedecor, George W. and William G. Cochran. 1972. *Statistical Methods*. Ames: Iowa State University Press.

Stewart, David W. and Prem N. Shamdasani. 1990. *Focus Groups: Theory and Practice.* Applied Social Research Methods Series 20. New York: Sage.

Stover, J. et al. 1995. "Impact of interventions on reducing the spread of HIV in Africa: Computer simulation applications." *African Journal of Medical Practice* 2.

Suchman, Edward A. 1967. *Evaluative Research: Principles and Practices in Public Services and Social Action Programs*. New York: Russell Sage Foundation.

Susser, M. 1996. "Some principles in study design for preventing HIV transmission: Rigor or reality." *American Journal of Public Health* 86(12).

UNAIDS. 2000. *National AIDS Programmes: A Guide to Monitoring and Evaluation.* Geneva: Joint United Nations Programme on HIV/ AIDS.

———. 2000. *Costing Guidelines for HIV Prevention.* Geneva: Joint United Nations Programme on HIV/AIDS.

United Nations Statistics Office. 1960. *A Short Manual on Sampling Studies in Methods*, Series F, No. 9. New York: United Nations.

United States General Accounting Office. 1992 (Revised in May). *Using Statistical Sampling* (GAO/PMED-10.1.6). Washington: GAO.

Van Dam, C. Johannes, Gina Dallabetta, and Peter Piot. 1999. "Prevention and control of sexually transmitted diseases in developing countries," in *Sexually Transmitted Diseases* (3rd ed.), ed. King Holmes et al. New York: McGraw Hill, 1,381-1,390.

Von Schoen Angerer, Tido et al. 2001. "Access and activism: The ethics of providing antiretroviral therapy in developing countries." *AIDS* 15 (Supplement 5): S81–S90.

Wawer, Maria et al. 1997. "Trends in HIV-1 prevalence may not reflect trends in incidence of mature epidemics: Data from the Rakai population-based cohort, Uganda." *AIDS* 11: 1,023–1,030.

Webb, Eugene J. et al. 1966. *Unobtrusive Measures: Non-Respective Research in the Social Sciences.* Chicago: Rand McNally.

Weber, Robert Philip. 1990. *Basic Content Analysis.* Thousand Oaks, CA: Sage.

Weiss, Carol H. 1972. *Evaluation Research: Methods for Assessing Program Effectiveness.* Englewood Cliffs, NJ: Prentice-Hall.

ADDITIONAL RESOURCES

Selected HIV/AIDS-Related Websites

www.unaids.org
Joint United Nations Programme on HIV/AIDS, a partnership of UNICEF, UNDP, UNFPA, UNDCP, ILO, UNESCO, WHO, World Bank.

www.aidsmap.com
Produced by NAM in collaboration with British HIV Association and International HIV/AIDS Alliance.

www.infoweb.org
An online library containing HIV/AIDS-related information.

www.iaen.org
International AIDS Economic Network: data, tools, and analysis for a compassionate, cost-effective response to the global epidemic.

www.hopkins-aids.edu
Johns Hopkins University AIDS Service.

www.nih.gov/od/oar/
National Institutes of Health (NIH) Office of AIDS Research.

http://sis.nlm.nih.gov/aids/
Guide to all NIH HIV/AIDS-related activities and information.

www.who.int/HIV-vaccines/
Joint WHO-UNAIDS HIV Vaccine Initiative.

www.who.int/HIV_AIDS/
World Health Organization Department of HIV/AIDS.

www.rho.org/html/hiv_aids.htm
Reproductive Health Outlook, produced by PATH.

www.usaid.gov/pop_health/aids/
United States Agency for International Aid, Department of Global Health Program for HIV/AIDS.

www.popcouncil.org/horizons
Population Council's Horizons Program.

www.statpages.net
Links to hundreds of websites that perform statistical calculations.

www.aegis.com
AIDS Education Global Information System.

www.undp.org/hiv
United Nations Development Programme, HIV/AIDS Section.

http://hivinsite.ucsf.edu/InSite
Comprehensive, current information on HIV treatment, prevention, and policy from the University of California–San Francisco (UCSF).

www.caps.ucsf.edu
Center for AIDS Prevention Studies at UCSF.

www.aids.harvard.edu/
  Harvard AIDS Institute is dedicated to conducting and catalyzing research to end the worldwide AIDS epidemic.

www.ama-assn.org/special/hiv/
  Journal of the American Medical Association HIV/AIDS Resource Center; includes in-depth reports, an online library, and treatment guidelines.

www.ama-assn.org/ama/pub/category/
  1944.html
  American Medical Association Section on HIV/AIDS.

www.census.gov/ipc/www/hivaidsn.html
  US Census Bureau HIV/AIDS Surveillance; includes surveillance database and selected developing country profiles.

www.cdc.gov/hiv/dhap.htm
  U.S. Centers for Disease Control and Prevention (CDC), Center for HIV/AIDS Prevention.

www.cdcnpin.org
  CDC National Prevention Information Network: U.S. reference, referral, and distribution service for information on HIV/AIDS, STDs, and tuberculosis.

www.aids-ed.org
  AIDS Education Training Centers, National Resource Center.

www.aidsinafrica.com
  Comprehensive, up-to-date information and news on AIDS in Africa.

http://www.measuredhs.com/hivdata
  Provides an easily accessible comprehensive source of information on HIV/AIDS indicators derived from sample surveys; allows the user to produce tables for specific countries by selected background characteristics.

Selected HIV/AIDS-Related Journals

AIDS
Official journal of the International AIDS Society.
www.aidsonline.com

AIDS and Behavior
Scientific exchange of information on the neurobehavioral factors in the initial spread, behavioral consequences, and social impact and response to HIV infection.
www.kluweronline.com/issn/1090-7165/

AIDS Care
Psychological and sociomedical aspects of HIV/AIDS.
www.tandf.co.uk/journals/titles/09540121.html

AIDS Education & Prevention: An Interdisciplinary Journal
Discusses models of AIDS education and prevention, and a wide range of public health, psychosocial, ethical, and public policy concerns related to HIV and AIDS.
www.guilford.com/cartscript.cgi?page=periodicals/jnai.htm

AIDS & Public Policy Journal
A peer-reviewed journal that seeks to advance knowledge of the social, political, ethical, and legal issues arising in public health and health policy as they relate to AIDS. APPJ is published quarterly.
www.upgbooks.com/appj/index.html

International Journal of STD & AIDS
Provides a clinically oriented forum for papers reporting on the investigation and treatment of STDs and HIV/AIDS.

www.roysocmed.ac.uk/pub/std.htm

Journal of Acquired Immune Deficiency Syndromes

Provides a synthesis of information on AIDS and human retrovirology from all relevant clinical and basic sciences. www.jaids.com

Journal of HIV/AIDS

A peer-reviewed journal of current therapies published by the National Medical Society. www.ccspublishing.com/j_aids.htm

Journal of Infectious Diseases

Includes articles on research from microbiology, immunology, epidemiology, and related disciplines. www.journals.uchicago.edu/JID/home.html

Sexually Transmitted Infections (formerly Genitourinary Medicine)

The oldest journal in the field dealing with issues of sexual health, sexually transmitted diseases, and HIV. www.sextransinf.com